Becoming a Chiropractor

Is chiropractic really the career for you?

First edition

Edited by Professor Christina Cunliffe
Co-edited by Jane Cooke

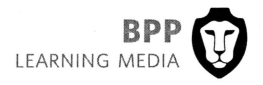

First edition 2013

ISBN 9781 4453 9724 5
e-ISBN 9781 4453 9733 7

British Library Cataloguing-in-Publication Data

A catalogue record for this book is available from the British Library

Published by

BPP Learning Media Ltd
BPP House, Aldine Place
London W12 8AA

www.bpp.com/health

Printed in the UK by
Ricoh
Ricoh House
Ullswater Crescent
Coulsdon
CR5 2HR

Your learning materials, published by BPP Learning Media Ltd, are printed on paper sourced from sustainable, managed forests.

The views expressed in this book are those of BPP Learning Media and not those of UCAS or any universities. BPP Learning Media are in no way associated with or endorsed by UCAS or any universities.

The contents of this book are intended as a guide and not professional advice. Although every effort has been made to ensure that the contents of this book are correct at the time of going to press, BPP Learning Media, makes no warranty that the information in this book is accurate or complete and accept no liability for any loss or damage suffered by any person acting or refraining from acting as a result of the material in this book.

Every effort has been made to contact the copyright holders of any material reproduced within this publication. If any have been inadvertently overlooked, BPP Learning Media will be pleased to make the appropriate credits in any subsequent reprints or editions.

BPP
LEARNING MEDIA

Contents

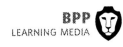

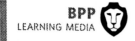

Free companion material

Readers can access additional companion material for free online.

To access companion material please visit:
www.bpp.com/freehealthresources.

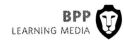

About the publisher

BPP Learning Media is dedicated to supporting aspiring professionals with top quality learning material. BPP Learning Media's commitment to success is shown by our record of quality, innovation and market leadership in paper-based and e-learning materials. BPP Learning Media's study materials are written by professionally-qualified specialists who know from personal experience the importance of top quality materials for success.

About the editors / contributors

Christina Cunliffe

Christina Cunliffe obtained her PhD from the University of Manchester, and is a graduate of the McTimoney College of Chiropractic in Abingdon. A member of the General Chiropractic Council, she sits on its Education Committee and is Chair of the Resource Management Committee. She is a Fellow of the College of Chiropractors, and currently holds the position of Treasurer on the College Council. She has been the Principal of the McTimoney College of Chiropractic based in Abingdon since 1998, and is a visiting lecturer at Oxford University, Oxford Brookes University and Warwick University Medical School. She maintains her practice in Oxfordshire.

Jane Cooke

Jane Cooke gained her first degree BSc (Hons) at the University of Manchester Institute of Science and Technology prior to commencing a career as an editor and writer of general reference books and, subsequently, CD-ROMs and websites. (Employers included Reader's Digest and Dorling Kindersley.) She then returned to college to study chiropractic. Jane has continued to write and edit articles about chiropractic and healthcare while practising chiropractic in London.

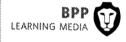

About the contributors

Maureen E Atkinson

Maureen Atkinson joined the Chiropractic Patients' Association in 1983 and became both Secretary and Treasurer in 1997. She was then invited to become a member of the newly formed Investigating Committee of the General Chiropractic Council (GCC) in 2002 and served for six years. In 2002 she was elected Chairman of the CPA and in that role represented the CPA on the Communications Strategy Advisory Group of the GCC and on the Council of the College of Chiropractors. Maureen was elected as the first Lay Fellow of the College of Chiropractors in 2008. In 2010 she was elected Secretary of Pro Chiropractic Europe to advance chiropractic treatment and the profession throughout the European community.

Peter Dixon

Peter Dixon graduated in 1984 from the Anglo-European College of Chiropractic (AECC) in Bournemouth, he then joined the British Chiropractic Association and was elected to their Council in 1986. He was President from 1994 to 1998 and then President of the European Chiropractors' Union from 2000 to 2004. Peter was on the Board of Governors of the AECC from 1992 to 1998 and Chairman from 1997 to 1998. He was elected to the council of the General Chiropractic Council (GCC) in 2001 and has been its chair since 2006.

Gayle Hoffman

Gayle Hoffman is currently Director of Admissions and Student Services at the McTimoney College of Chiropractic, and she previously held the same position at the New Zealand College of Chiropractic. After a successful career in sales and marketing in New York City, her love of chiropractic prompted a change of direction and she is now able to bring her previous skills to bear in her current role.

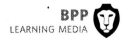

Michael B Bennett

Throughout his career Michael has lectured for many of the leading UK training establishments including the Anglo European College of Chiropractic, British School of Osteopathy, British College of Osteopathic Medicine, McTimoney College of Chiropractic, European School of Osteopathy, London Foot Hospital, London School of Osteopathy, Oxford Brookes, International College of Oriental Medicine, Brighton University and others. He has spoken at the Society of Chiropodists & Podiatrist annual conferences in Harrogate and Glasgow and has run numerous CPD courses both in his own right and on behalf of the College of Chiropractors, the British Osteopathic Association and the Society of Chiropodists & Podiatrists.

Valerie S Pennacchio

Val Pennacchio has been an educator in chiropractic for over 30 years in the USA, New Zealand and the UK. Over the years her teaching subjects have been highly varied and have included histology, X-ray analysis, pathology and clinical reasoning and also the philosophy and history of chiropractic in the context of its fit with modern healthcare. Val has also been at the coalface with students as they interact with patients applying their academic learning in real-life clinical practice.

Mary Young

Mary Young has spent most of her life in education one way or another, training as a riding instructor between school and university, and then becoming involved in undergraduate teaching as well as engaging in graduate study. She found chiropractic thanks to a veterinary referral when her dog was suffering and the immediate improvement achieved by the treatment was so persuasive that she decided to investigate the training process. Five years and a lot of financial and logistical juggling later, she is about to enter her final clinic year.

Gill Amos

Gill Amos obtained her degree in Applied Physics from Lanchester Polytechnic and spent fifteen years as a technical writer for a large software company in the south of England. After graduating as a chiropractor, she went on to gain her MSc Chiropractic (Small Animals).

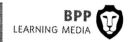

Gill is a Fellow of the College of Chiropractors and has held the position of Director of Continuing Professional Development on the College Council. She is in private practice in Berkshire where she runs a multi-disciplinary clinic for both people and small animals.

Rob Finch

Rob Finch trained as a biologist in the 1980s and completed his PhD in biotechnology at the University of Nottingham in 1991. He researched and lectured in the field of biotechnology for a number of years, publishing more than 20 academic papers and book chapters and directing education in applied biological sciences, before retraining in medical education at the University of Sheffield. Following a five-year period at the Royal College of Obstetricians and Gynaecologists, where he was Head of Education, Rob took up his current post as Chief Executive of the College of Chiropractors in 2003. His particular interests include effectiveness of Continuing Professional Development, service quality and patient safety.

Matthew Bennett

Matthew Bennett has worked in several practices around the UK and in New Zealand. He has visited many other practices looking for the ingredients that make these clinics happy and successful places to work. In his Brighton clinic he has worked closely with more than 20 new graduates assisting in their postgraduate training and development. He lectures regularly to audiences of chiropractors on business management and marketing and also runs a consultancy for chiropractors wanting to get the most out of their practice. As well as training new graduates he also trains other chiropractors to become trainers in their own right. Matthew is a Fellow of the College of Chiropractors and Vice President of the British Chiropractic Association.

Marisa Pinnock

Marisa Pinnock as been a chiropractor in private practice since 1996. She holds a master's degree in Animal Chiropractic and is Chair of the College of Chiropractors Animal Chiropractic Faculty, Director of College of Chiropractors CPD, past Member of the General Chiropractic Council, Education Committee and Investigating Committee, and past Chair MCA Animal Group. She lectures and examines chiropractic students and regularly speaks at courses and national conferences.

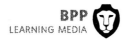

Richard Skippings

Richard Skippings graduated from the Anglo-European College of Chiropractic in 1985. He became a Certified Chiropractic Sports Physician in 1991, gained a Post Graduate Diploma in Sports Medicine from Sheffield University in 2009 and was awarded the International Chiropractic Sports Science Diploma also in 2009. He is an Honorary Life member of the British Chiropractic Sports Council, a member of the Fédèration Internationale de Chiropratique du Sport and a member of its Board of Education. He is a Specialist Fellow and the Chair of the College of Chiropractors Faculty for Sport and Exercise. He is also a member of the British Association of Sport & Exercise Medicine.

Adrian Hunnisett

Whilst working as a biomedical scientist, Adrian Hunnisett graduated in Human Biology from Oxford Brookes University and then gained his MPhil and PhD by research from the same university. He has a varied career within healthcare in the NHS and private medical sectors with posts as varied as a biomedical scientist, Principal Biochemist, GP Business Manager and, most recently, Head of Clinical Research at a major UK teaching hospital. Adrian has also been an external examiner at the University of Middlesex and acts as a research consultant to a clinical nutrition college in Berkshire. He holds a Fellowship qualification in clinical biochemistry with the Institute of Biomedical Scientists, is a Member of the Institute of Clinical Research and an accredited Chartered Scientist. Currently he is employed as Research Director at McTimoney College of Chiropractic in Oxfordshire.

Foreword by Quentin Willson

First things first. I'm not a user of alternative therapies or medicines. I'm a bloke, and most of us don't do that new age stuff. Plus I'm an alpha male, skidding breathlessly through life like Alice's white rabbit concerned only with the things I can see touch and prove empirically. Which makes my view of chiropractic particularly significant. You see, two things happened in my life to make me understand that chiropractic definitely and absolutely works. No doubt about it. This then, is the unimpeachable testimony of the man who didn't want to believe.

The first defining moment came, when out of desperation, I took my five-year-old son Max to Deidre Edwards in Stratford-on-Avon – a McTimoney chiropractor, specialising in children. Max was on the autistic spectrum with Asperger's and wouldn't sleep, eat or behave properly. My wife and I had suffered five years of abject, sleepless misery and tried literally everything. We'd been to every health professional and then some, but nothing ever seemed to work. Our expectations were low but we thought we'd give the off-beat idea of some chiropractic adjustments a try. That very same night Max slept 12 hours straight for the first time in his life. Weekly visits followed and his behaviour, sleep patterns, sense of taste and smell and eating slowly normalised. Soon he began to regularly articulate that his neck was stiff and he needed to see Deidre. The change in his personality, happiness and abilities was nothing short of staggering. Eight years later he's now in a mainstream school, a flourishing teenager and coping admirably with life. He still has his chiropractic adjustments and still tells us when he needs a top up. (See Chapter 8, *Routine or variety?*.)

The second seminal moment came when my wife, Michaela, was diagnosed with a damaged vertebra that had flared up from an old water skiing accident. We'd tried doctors, osteopaths and spinal specialists and we were all set to have an operation involving an incision in the throat, moving her voice box to one side and inserting a steel plate in her spine. Desolated and desperate we again visited our chiropractor. And again that miraculous change started to happen. The adjustments took several weeks to improve her mobility and reduce the pain but within two months Michaela was almost back to normal. Like Max, she still has her regular adjustments but the pain has gone and she never had to suffer that awful, invasive surgery.

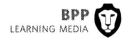

Now the whole family goes to our chiropractor. A kind of 'weekly tune up'. And even I, the rank unbeliever, can feel the difference. If it was up to me I'd make every child have adjustments from birth and commission a massive medical field trial to establish and understand the effects. But since you're reading this book you want to understand and that's the first step. Take it from me, the chiropractic advocate who has absolutely no agenda at all, it's a remarkable therapy that society really should know much, much more about.

Quentin Willson
British TV presenter and motoring expert

Shining a light on your future career path

The process of researching and identifying a career that you are most suited to can be a somewhat daunting process, but the rewards of following a career that truly engages you should not be underestimated. Deciding on your future career path should be viewed as a fun and extremely satisfying process that, if done correctly, will benefit you greatly.

Carefully considering a short list of future career options and what each one will offer you will help you to make a truly informed decision. Although it is perfectly acceptable to change career direction at a later date, reviewing the options open to you now will help to ensure that you are satisfied with your career from the outset.

I first began mentoring aspiring professionals eight years ago when it was clear that many individuals were not gaining access to the careers guidance they required. It was with this in mind that I embarked on publishing our *Becoming a* series of books, to provide help, support and clear insight into career choices. I hope that this book will help you to make an informed decision as to what career you are most suited to, your strengths and your aspirations.

I would like to take this opportunity to wish you the very best of luck with identifying your future career and hope that you pass on some of the gems of wisdom that you acquire along the way, to those who follow in your footsteps.

Matt Green
Series Editor – *Becoming a* series
Director of Professional Development
BPP University College of Professional Studies

Chapter 1

The journey begins!

Christina Cunliffe

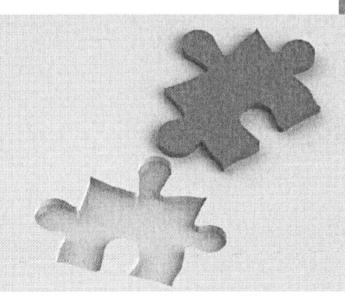

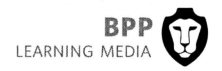

Introduction

If the title of this chapter gives you a thrill of excitement then you are ready to put your foot on the path to what all chiropractors consider to be the best career in the world!

Becoming a chiropractor is a very personal journey. Perhaps you have been helped by a chiropractor, or maybe a friend or a member of your family has told you about their experiences, and this has got you thinking about whether or not chiropractic is the career for you. It may be that you are interested in health generally and are exploring a number of different options. The fact that you are reading this book though means that you are seriously considering either embarking on a new career, or a change in career, and want to know how to go about it and what the implications might be.

My own journey began when I was helped by a chiropractor. The GP told me that the tingling in my leg could be the start of multiple sclerosis but he wouldn't do any tests until it became worse. A friend suggested I went to a local chiropractor who examined me and said the problem was with my lumbar spine. She was right; she adjusted me, the tingling cleared up and never returned. That day a seed was planted in my mind and over the next few years it grew until I knew that this was something that I really wanted to do.

That's when I started to question myself: do I really want to leave a very good job? What will I be able to earn as a chiropractor? Will I be able to maintain the same lifestyle? What will my friends and family think? How can I fit in my studies? Can I even learn to do this amazing thing that my chiropractor does? I soon realised though that self-doubt was the only thing that was holding me back, and I applied to chiropractic college the very next day. Looking back I can say that the journey has always been interesting, full of variety, challenging and rewarding. Becoming a chiropractor was the best decision I ever made in my life. I hope it will be for you too.

> 'Your time is limited, so don't waste it living someone else's life. Don't be trapped by dogma – which is living with the results of other people's thinking. Don't let the noise of others' opinions drown out your own inner voice.' (Steve Jobs, 2005)

The purpose of this book is to provide you with more information about chiropractic, but it also aims to offer you different perspectives that might help you as you make your decision. It starts off by telling you a little bit about chiropractic and what chiropractors do. The art of manipulation can be traced back to early cave drawings and was used extensively by the Greeks, but chiropractic itself was founded in

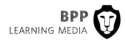

1895 in Davenport, Iowa, USA. Named from the Greek 'chiropractikos' meaning done by hand, chiropractic has grown and developed into a well-recognised profession around the world. There are many chiropractic colleges around the world, including the UK, and new colleges are springing up all the time.

It is a primary care profession regulated by an Act of Parliament in the UK and is quickly establishing itself as a mainstream healthcare provider. Because of this status, chiropractors are respected members of the community in which they work, and if you choose to join the profession you will find that this brings with it certain responsibilities in your personal as well as your professional life. This is the price, if you like, of being a 'professional', and as a health professional the safety and care of your patients is paramount.

It would be very easy to just talk about chiropractic and chiropractors, but the patient's perspective is the most valuable of all. Thousands of patients seek chiropractic care every day and they do so knowing that they will have to pay for the services provided. Working with patients is what makes this career so varied and interesting. The majority of chiropractors work in general practice seeing a wide range of people from all walks of life. The people who walk through your clinic door may be young or old, sporty or sedentary, in pain or with a disability, or making a lifestyle choice for health and wellbeing. They may come alone, with their carers, or as part of a family group. Whoever they are, they will trust you, not only to give their body the very best of care, but often with personal and private details of their lives.

> In the USA there are more visits to complementary health practitioners than medical doctors every year, and considering that patients there have to pay for whichever form of care they choose, the implication is that they are not making a choice based on financial reasons, but on the value they place on the care they receive. In the UK our National Health Service is free, and so it is even more significant that people still choose to pay for private chiropractic care in their many thousands.

You will not be able to help everyone, of course, and knowing when to refer to others is an important element of working within a multidisciplinary team of fellow health professionals who also have the patient's best interests at heart. This team may work in the same clinic as you or they may be located in your vicinity, but either way you will be part of a network of individuals who will each bring their own unique skills and experience into the mix and work together for the best clinical outcome.

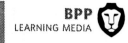

As you will have full responsibility for the people under your care, the training is necessarily rigorous. In many ways the training is equivalent to that of a medical doctor, as chiropractors have to be able to recognise any underlying problems that might indicate referral for further tests or evaluations. Although chiropractors do not prescribe drugs, you will learn about pharmacology, as many of your patients will be taking over-the-counter or prescribed medications and you will need to know about side-effects and how the drugs may affect the patient.

The practice of chiropractic and medicine are very different, however. You will learn more anatomy and biomechanics on a chiropractic programme, for example, because this essential knowledge will inform how you adjust the spine. Obviously, you will also learn a variety of chiropractic techniques and patient management skills. Because chiropractors mostly work in private practice, unlike medical doctors, you will be taught how to establish and grow your own business as well.

You will earn a good living as a chiropractor, but many chiropractors do not regard this as their main reason for working. The profession's primary motivation is to help patients manage their lifestyle and health, and if you do that well then your business will grow as a result. In fact, your motivation is probably one of the most important factors overall – why is it that you are thinking about becoming a chiropractor? It will certainly be something your interviewers will want to explore when you attend an interview.

Even though you are just considering embarking on your chiropractic journey, it won't be long before you realise that this is just the start of your lifelong learning! All chiropractors undertake annual continuing professional development courses that stimulate their thinking and enhance their skills base, but many enrol on postgraduate programmes that give them additional qualifications in specialist areas like sports, paediatrics or animal care. There is no career structure as such within the profession, but you can decide to focus on a particular area of practice, go into teaching or research, get involved in the development of the profession, or any combination of the above. It is entirely up to you to determine how you direct your future.

"Good Luck, this is the first day of the rest of your life." These are the words my mum used when I left for my first day at chiropractic college nearly five years ago. **New chiropractor on graduation day**

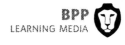

You are the only one who can decide what kind of chiropractor you want to become, and you will probably find that the idea you have now of your perfect practice will evolve as you progress through your training. The more knowledge you gain and the different perspectives you absorb will all inform your development as an individual, and therefore as a student chiropractor. It may not surprise you to know that this process will continue even when you have been practising for many years because, just as the profession is growing and changing, so will you.

You will not be alone on your journey. In your class you will find people just like you who are excited about becoming a chiropractor, and you will be taught by staff who are chiropractors and who have been trained themselves in similar circumstances. A chiropractic programme is a lot tougher than many other degrees you can enrol on, but the sense of community that you will find, and the friendships that you will make, will last a lifetime.

Everything you learn during your chiropractic programme, from your first lecture on how the body works to your final day in the student clinic putting it all into practice, will prepare you to start on your chosen career and become the chiropractor you want to be. From your very first day, consider yourself as a 'professional in training' rather than a student, because that's when you start to become a chiropractor.

Your future is in your hands!

References

Stanford Report (2005) *'You've Got to Find What You Love' Job says. Prepared text of the Commencement Address Delivered by Steve Jobs, CEO of Apple Computer and of Pixar Animation Studios, on June 12, 2005.*
[Online] Available at: http://news.stanford.edu/news/2005/june15/jobs-061505.html [Accessed 29 July 2012]

Chapter 2

What do chiropractors do?

Jane Cooke

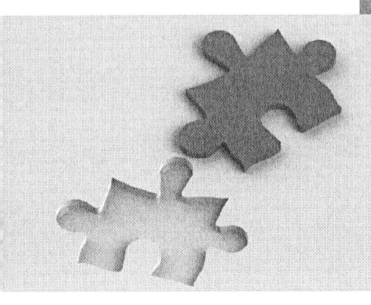

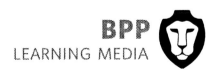

Chiropractic is primarily concerned with the diagnosis, treatment, prevention and rehabilitation of common neuro-musculoskeletal complaints ('neuro' referring to the nervous system and 'musculoskeletal' to the framework of bones and muscles that support the body). There is an emphasis on non-invasive manual treatments and the restoration of optimum function to the body. Chiropractors take a holistic and patient-centred approach to their practices, using a variety of manual techniques plus other modalities, such as soft tissue therapy and exercise regimes. The profession recognises and is involved in the development of an increasing body of evidence-based research supporting chiropractic.

Definition

Holistic health is a concept that is widely accepted in medical practice. The holistic premise is that all aspects of a patient's needs, including physical, psychological and social, should be taken into account and viewed as a whole during assessment and treatment planning. In physical terms, chiropractors tend to check the whole body (rather than just the 'bit that hurts'). If one part of the body (eg the knee) is painful, it is likely that another part of the body (eg the pelvis) is compensating and needs attention too.

More than just 'cracking backs'

Chiropractors provide care for patients of all ages who present with a range of acute (short-term) and chronic (longer-term) conditions. As well helping with pain management, injuries and rehabilitation, chiropractors will look at a patient's clinical picture in the long term: offering advice, for example, on self-help, exercise, diet and lifestyle. Practitioners take an integrated approach to the health needs of their patients, considering not only their presenting physical condition, but also their medical history, lifestyle (sleep, diet, stress levels and so on), and social factors, for example, how much support they have at home. Chiropractors provide care and continuing support by reducing pain and disability, restoring best possible function to patients and by preventing future episodes of pain.

Chiropractors place an emphasis on manual treatments, involving the precise handling or moving of parts of the body into optimal position (this is generally known as 'adjustment' or 'manipulation'). The treatment options available to a qualified chiropractor, however, are wide and not limited solely to adjustment. A variety of techniques are used to help patients, many of which do not involve the 'cracking' so often associated with chiropractic (and which has been known to put off some prospective patients). See Chapter 11.

Significantly, chiropractors do not just treat backs; they can often help manage neck pain and headache stemming from the neck, migraine, dizziness, a variety problems in the extremities and many other conditions – some of which have been researched more extensively than others.

First-hand experience

The best way of finding out what a chiropractor does is probably to experience or observe one in action (bearing in mind that chiropractors' clinics and techniques can vary). You may consider attending a clinic as a patient. You do not need to be in pain to see a chiropractor as the treatment can rectify subtle problems that you might notice only after the minor niggles have abated post-treatment. Remember too that chiropractic can help prevent pain occurring in the first place because, in many cases, pain will only arise after your body has struggled to correct itself for some time already. Pain is simply the body's signal telling you that something is wrong, and it will shout louder and louder until you hear it.

Most chiropractors should be willing to allow you to observe if you show a keen interest in pursuing this career, although this may be harder for sole practitioners to accommodate. Ideally, you will visit a large, multi-practitioner clinic and, perhaps, someone working from a home clinic – then you can fill in the gaps with your vision of the perfect practice for you. You will be in the happy position, once qualified, of deciding for yourself how you wish to practise as long as you adhere to the General Chiropractic Council (GCC) Code of Practice and Standard of Proficiency.

The GCC Code of Practice and Standard of Proficiency

The General Chiropractic Council's Code of Practice and Standard of Proficiency (CoP and SoP) sets out the quality of care that patients are entitled to receive from chiropractors. The standards apply to all chiropractors practising in the UK, whatever their employment status or environment in which they practise. The full document is available from the GCC website but, essentially, the CoP and SoP cover the following topics:

The Code of Practice stipulates that you must

- Respect the dignity, individuality and privacy of patients
- Respect the rights of patients to be involved in decisions about their healthcare
- Justify public trust and confidence by being honest and trustworthy
- Provide a good standard of practice and care
- Protect patients and colleagues from risk of harm
- Cooperate with colleagues from your own and other professions

The Standard of Proficiency covers the following

- Practice arrangements
- Assessing the health and health needs of patients
- The provision of chiropractic care

To find a practitioner in your area, you can use the search facilities on the various chiropractic association websites. Another good way of finding a chiropractor is via a word-of-mouth recommendation, as chiropractic is a very personal approach to healthcare. Many experienced chiropractors continue to rely on word-of-mouth referrals to maintain or expand their practices.

Top tip

Finding a chiropractor

To find a chiropractor in your area, you can refer to the GCC website. You can also find chiropractors via the professional associations either directly or through their websites and adverts in the local Yellow Pages: the British Chiropractic Association (BCA); the McTimoney Chiropractic Association (MCA); the United Chiropractic Association (UCA) and the Scottish Chiropractic Association (SCA). Consider asking around for a recommendation first and do not jump to conclusions: the chiropractic profession is regulated by statute but affords flexibility in practice.

What happens at a chiropractic consultation?

The types of chiropractic intervention will be dictated, to a large extent, by the presenting complaint, and one of your first tasks as a chiropractor in clinic will be to take a full clinical case history. Some problems of the musculoskeletal system, for example, are caused by accidents, lack of exercise and / or poor posture, illness or everyday wear and tear. You will look for vital clues in your history taking, a bit like a private detective, including the location, duration and nature of pain, any aggravating or alleviating factors, past history of trauma, previous or current illnesses or medical interventions, medication and family history. You can then start to piece together both the obvious and less obvious causes behind a patient's symptoms.

> 'Neuro-musculoskeletal pain rarely has one single cause and I have always found that the detective work involved in making your provisional differential diagnosis is one the most interesting parts of the job.'

Following the history taking, you will carry out a physical examination – using sight and touch (or 'palpation'). This examination will include neurological and orthopaedic tests if needed and you may require an image of the patient's spine or other joints or further diagnostic tests. Your first concern will be to find out what is causing the problem and whether it falls within the remit of chiropractic care. So, you will routinely check for signs and symptoms of any serious conditions that require referral to the patient's GP or to hospital for emergency care. In this way you will provide a valuable 'screening' service for your patients while reassuring doctors that chiropractors understand their obligations to refer when necessary. All this must take place before you discuss your findings with the patient and gain their consent to your proposed treatment.

BPP LEARNING MEDIA

Case study

Mrs P was a factory worker in her mid-forties who suffered with excessive back pain from regular heavy lifting. Chiropractic every two to three months, coupled with home rehabilitation exercises, kept her well. On one visit to her chiropractor he noticed a black mole on her back, about a centimetre in diameter, dark and slightly raised. It looked normal, but the chiropractor decided to measure it and repeat the measurement in six months. In that time it grew 1mm, so she was referred to her GP, who asked a dermatologist to take a look. The specialist did not think it was serious but decided to remove the mole anyway and, on biopsy, it was found to be a malignant melanoma. A further deep excision was carried out two weeks later. The surgeon said that finding the malignancy early and its radical removal had probably saved Mrs P's life.

What is the General Chiropractic Council?

The GCC is a UK-wide statutory body with regulatory powers, established by the Chiropractors Act 1994. It has three main duties:

- To protect the public by establishing and operating a scheme of statutory regulation for chiropractors, similar to the arrangements that cover other health professionals

- To set the standards of chiropractic education, conduct and practice

- To ensure the development of the profession of chiropractic, using a model of continuous improvement in practice

First things first

To work as a chiropractor in the UK you must register with the GCC, and to register you must have completed a university degree programme recognised by the Council. Students in the UK typically study for four years to gain their chiropractic qualification. For detailed information about the accredited degree programmes, see Chapter 6. The GCC promotes equality of opportunity but all graduates must be able to show that they have met all the learning outcomes of the programme of study and can meet the standard for chiropractic practice. There is a guide published by the GCC for those with a disability or health condition, which provides useful examples to help you with your decision-making: *A Guide for Disabled People* (2010) – see Useful resources.

The GCC continues to assess and assure the quality of education at the three chiropractic colleges that have attained suitable accreditation: the Anglo-European College of Chiropractic; the McTimoney College of Chiropractic; and the Welsh Institute of Chiropractic.

Freedom in practice

You will read much about the rigorous undergraduate training and stringent requirements for chiropractic registration, but never lose sight of the freedom that a chiropractic career can bring you. Most chiropractic graduates will enter into private practice because there is limited scope for chiropractors to operate within the National Health Service (NHS) – a situation that may well change as the NHS authorities review their contracts with private health providers. This paucity of free care exists despite the fact that chiropractic care is included in the *Musculoskeletal Services Framework* published by the Department of Health and the National Institute for Health and Clinical Excellence (NICE) Guidelines – see Useful resources.

Time is on your side

'As a chiropractor, you are likely to have more contact time with a patient compared with a GP, for example, and time is often what a chiropractic patient needs most, especially if a condition is chronic or complex. You will have time to find out the causes of a problem, rather just treating the symptoms. This is the type of patient-centred care that people are increasingly demanding and of which (in theory, at least) the NHS is aiming to increase provision.'

General Practitioners (GPs) have relatively limited resources at their disposal with regard to treating musculoskeletal pain. Yet around a quarter of all patients attend a GP's surgery with this type of problem. Drugs, physiotherapy or, as a last resort, surgery, may be all the doctor can offer to a patient with persistent musculoskeletal pain. GPs will routinely refer chronic back pain patients for physiotherapy, for example, partly because GPs can easily refer to physiotherapists on the NHS and because the two professions have worked alongside one another for many years. The physiotherapist though may only have a ten-minute appointment available for the patient in six weeks' time, after which point manual intervention can become less effective, according to the NICE guidelines.

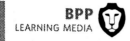

The causes of neuro-musculoskeletal pain are often complicated and cannot be fully addressed in ten-minute windows. Conditions, such as severe lower back pain, unremitting headache and degenerative arthritis can be debilitating, depressing and, in the long term, they undermine an individual's lifestyle and ambitions. This is where you can step in as a caring and highly motivated new chiropractor!

Top tip

All the major insurance companies cover chiropractic, sometimes (but not always) following a GP referral. You can sign up to most insurance companies' practitioner lists as soon as you are registered with the GCC – apart from BUPA, which requires you to fulfil specific criteria before they will accept you as a consultant provider.

Letting medics know what you do

As a newly qualified chiropractor, you may find that GPs and other medical professionals, including orthopaedic consultants, have differing perceptions of chiropractic. Some are familiar with the profession and will readily arrange a private chiropractic referral. Others may be dubious; often because they do not understand what chiropractic is or they have misperceptions about what chiropractic involves. Osteopathy is more familiar to many doctors, having been established in the UK for longer and also, perhaps, because the osteopathic profession has been more effective in communicating its collective message.

The good news is that the study of integrative, or complementary, medicine (including chiropractic) is now taught in undergraduate modules in many medical schools. Most doctors are keen to know that there are other options for their 'heart sink' chronic pain patients whom they have been unable to help. They need to know what chiropractors can do and to be assured that we belong to a fully regulated profession with extremely high educational standards and that we acknowledge and implement evidence-based practice.

The best way to convince a local GP that chiropractic works is to treat them yourself. Alternatively, many practice managers will agree for you to give a presentation to your local practice, and this is where the presentation skills that you have honed at college will prove invaluable. Be prepared and undaunted: there is good evidence-based research that supports chiropractic (see Chapter 16) and doctors rely on such research to direct the treatment of their patients.

Top tip

Take special note of the 2009 guidelines issued by the National Institute for Health and Clinical Excellence (NICE): *Early Management of Persistent Non-specific Low Back Pain*. GPs have been actively encouraged to refer to chiropractors by the British Medical Association (BMA) for the treatment of lower back pain, so you can use these guidelines as a starting point to demonstrate to doctors what other conditions chiropractic can help with.

NICE guidelines for management of low back pain

The National Institute for Health and Clinical Excellence (NICE) produces guidelines for healthcare professionals and others to ensure that the care they provide is of the best possible quality and offers the best value for money. The institute evaluates evidence-based research and makes recommendations for the most effective ways to prevent, diagnose and treat disease and ill health. Guidelines for low back pain were issued in 2009 and concern the treatment of people with persistent low back pain within the NHS in England and Wales. The document recommends that doctors should consider offering a course of manual therapy, including spinal manipulation, in cases of non-specific low back pain that has lasted for more than six weeks but less than 12 months.

Chiropractic and osteopathy

You will probably be asked the question, 'What is the difference between a chiropractor and an osteopath?' repeatedly as a student and a chiropractor. There is no simple answer. Happily, most people can now discern the difference between chiropractic and chiropody, (which was not so even five to ten years ago)! It may be helpful to look at the two professions from an historical perspective.

The genesis of chiropractic is commonly attributed to a consultation in the USA in 1895. Daniel David (DD) Palmer, known as the discoverer of chiropractic, placed his hands on an 'irregular protrusion of the spine of a patient and, with a thrust, reduced the irregularity' (Palmer, 1910). As a result, the patient claimed, not only that his back pain disappeared but his hearing was restored. DD Palmer, and subsequently many other followers, continued to practise 'chiropractic' in spite of opposition from allopathic, or orthodox, healthcare providers. DD Palmer maintained that chiropractic was a more natural approach to healing that drew upon

BPP LEARNING MEDIA

the body's own recuperative powers. Rather than just recognising the effects of disease, he wanted to address the underlying causes through the new healing art he discovered.

A little earlier, in 1874, Andrew Taylor Still, the founder of osteopathy, suffered from frequent headaches with nausea at the age of ten. He constructed a rope swing between two trees and lay down using the rope for a swinging pillow, after which he wrote, 'Soon I became easy and went to sleep, got up in a little while with headache all gone' (Still, 1910). He subsequently recognised that disease could have its origins in slight anatomical deviation from normal and set about proving that he could restore health by treating the human body with his hands using 'osteopathy'. Andrew Still understood that the human body is composed of many parts, all intimately related as a whole, and that optimal health is possible only when the body functions in harmony.

The historical and philosophical overlaps are obvious and yet, over time, comparisons between the two professions have become muddied. Differences between chiropractic and osteopathy can only be presented as generalisations. Both professions essentially adhere to the same principals of holistic healthcare, but there are philosophical differences and different techniques are employed in practice. Much depends on the individual practitioner and the presenting case, and it is good to remember that a patient may remain loyal to you because of your personal attributes (for example, communication skills, time allocation and sympathetic approach) more than the practical modalities that you employ in clinic, which can be equally effective in the right hands.

Chiropractic and osteopathy are both statutorily regulated and governed by general councils.
There is an overlap between the disciplines, and a significant portion of the workload is similar.
It can be said that chiropractors rely more on adjustment, or manipulation, which affects the nervous system, while osteopaths traditionally may focus on soft tissue rehabilitation and blood flow.
Many chiropractors tend to use more diagnostic procedures, such as X-rays and MRI scans.
Both professions aim to relieve pain and restore optimum function to the patient.

Table 2.1: Chiropractic and osteopathy – similarities and differences

Singh v the British Chiropractic Association

While searching for information about chiropractic on the internet, you will invariably come across references to a court case: *Simon Singh v the British Chiropractic Association (BCA) 2009–2010.* This case ultimately contested the issue of freedom of speech rather than the validity of chiropractic. It is important to know that the debate was essentially about libel law, and that an agreement was reached not to pursue the case due to the cost. The case was closed before any evidence concerning chiropractic was actually examined in court. This high-profile case did set precedents for the reform of libel law in the UK, but it did not disprove or cast doubt on the efficacy of chiropractic.

2: What do chiropractors do?

Chapter summary

As we have seen in this chapter, chiropractic is more than just 'cracking backs' – it is a fulfiling and flexible profession. Moreover, there has never been a better time to become a chiropractor. It has been a long journey for the profession – through higher education and statutory regulation – but now there is a greater understanding of the work chiropractors do due to better communication and a greater cohesion among the chiropractic organisations. Thousands of new patients visit a chiropractor each year in the UK. Around 150,000 new patients consult a McTimoney Chiropractor each year, for example, and these are the graduates of just one college. These numbers are increasing due to good treatment success rates and very high levels of patient satisfaction. Several studies, including the Gallup Study and the Harris Poll, have found that chiropractic patients are *highly* likely to be *very* satisfied with their treatment... and a satisfied customer makes for a happy working life.

Key points

- Chiropractors diagnose, treat, rehabilitate and help prevent common neuro-musculoskeletal complaints.

- Practitioners take an holistic, patient-centred approach to the needs of their patients.

- A variety of techniques are used with an emphasis on non-invasive manual intervention, notably adjustment or manipulation.

- Before treatment begins, a clinical history is taken and a physical examination, including any necessary tests, is carried out.

- A good way to understand what a chiropractor does is to observe one in clinic.

- Chiropractors must adhere to strict codes of practice, but they can enjoy flexibility, eg time spent in clinic and techniques used, once qualified.

- An important part of a chiropractor's job is communicating with other healthcare professionals.

Useful resources

Backcare (charity): www.backcare.org.uk

British Chiropractic Association: www.chiropractic-uk.co.uk

Department of Health: www.dh.gov.uk

GCC: *Guide for Disabled People*:
www.gcc-uk.org/page.cfm?page_id=42

General Chiropractic Council: www.gcc-uk.org

McTimoney Chiropractic Association: www.mctimoneychiropractic.org

NICE guidelines for management of low back pain:
www.nice.org.uk/CG88

Scottish Chiropractic Association: www.sca-chiropractic.org

United Chiropractic Association: www.united-chiropractic.org

References

Palmer, DD (1910) *The Science, Art and Philosophy of Chiropractic.* Portland, Oregon: Portland Printing House Company.

Still, AT (1910 & 1992) *Osteopathy: Research and Practice.* Seattle, Washington: Eastland Press Inc.

BPP
LEARNING MEDIA

Chapter 3

Chiropractic from the patients' perspective

Maureen E Atkinson

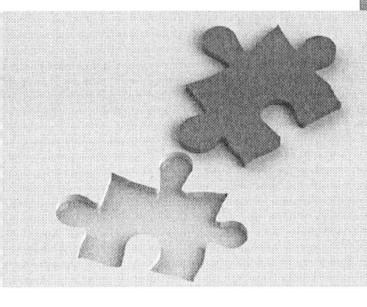

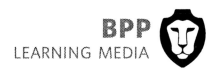

Without patients you will not have a practice. Patients are the reason that you become a chiropractor and become motivated to try to help them in whatever way you can. Patients' interests are looked after in a number of different ways, and you will find it useful to know about the various organisations and groups that support patients once you are in practice.

The Chiropractic Patients' Association

The Chiropractic Patients' Association (CPA) is a registered charity and owes its existence to grateful patients. These patients have been so indebted to their chiropractors for changing their lives that they have wanted other people to benefit too. Hence the CPA's remit to increase public awareness of the benefits of chiropractic treatment, to make it more available through the NHS and to support chiropractic research and education. The CPA is recognised as the voice of chiropractic patients by the General Chiropractic Council (GCC), and their lay members work with the Council on a number of the committees.

CPA membership

A tri-annual magazine, *Back Chat,* is published by the CPA and distributed free of charge to all chiropractic clinics. Contributions in the form of case studies and professional experiences from chiropractors, patients and students are encouraged, as well as news from the chiropractic colleges and associations. Many chiropractic clinics support the CPA by giving discounts to members and by displaying their information leaflets.

College of Chiropractors Lay Partnership Group

The College of Chiropractors (CoC) is the postgraduate college of the chiropractic profession (see Chapter 12) not to be confused with the undergraduate training colleges where you gain your chiropractic education (see Chapter 6). The Lay Partnership Group (LPG) was started with the specific purpose of ensuring that patients' voices were heard. Led by lay members (non-chiropractors), the LPG designed and sponsored the College's Patient Partnership Quality Mark (PPQM). This is an annual award given to chiropractic clinics that have shown excellence in meeting and exceeding patients' expectations in their quality of care.

The College believes that chiropractic services should be centred on the users of those services, namely chiropractic patients. It supports the delivery of services that are flexible and responsive to patients' needs, acknowledging them as partners in their own care. This view is endorsed by the Lay Partnership Group, which is a forum that provides a patient and public viewpoint with regard to college business and which develops initiatives to support patient advocacy. The LPG has a number of patient and public representatives, including the Chairman of the Chiropractic Patients' Association, as well as chiropractors who work with the group to provide professional advice.

Top tip

The Patient Partnership Quality Mark (PPQM) and the Clinical Management Quality Mark (CMQM) are awarded in recognition of excellence in terms of meeting patients' expectations. Once in practice, you should consider applying for these awards to demonstrate your commitment to quality patient care.

Patient Partnership Quality Mark (PPQM)

In 2006, the LPG launched a new quality mark for chiropractic practices, intended to recognise excellence in terms of meeting patient expectations. Chiropractic practices are required to demonstrate that they meet patient expectations in a wide range of areas, as identified by the lay members of the LPG, including the following:

- Accessibility
- Booking systems and out-of-hours cover
- Cleanliness and safety
- Privacy
- Communication
- Patient education
- Record keeping
- Other forms of care offered

As a chiropractor, you will be encouraged to apply for the PPQM to demonstrate your commitment to quality patient care. You will also be invited to explain how you undertake other activities to meet patient expectations in ways not envisaged by the LPG. Applications, which need to be supported by relevant evidence, are then considered by an LPG-appointed panel and judged on the form submitted, although the panel reserves the right to check the veracity of statements made. Each application is considered on its own merit regardless of the size of the practice.

Clinical Management Quality Mark (CMQM)

A second quality mark, the Clinical Management Quality Mark, was launched in 2008-9 to complement the PPQM. This award recognises excellence in terms of operating within a structured and managed clinical environment. If you apply for this important quality mark, you will have to demonstrate excellence in a range of areas, including: clinical audit, risk management, incident reporting, outcome measurement and patient satisfaction – all of which are expected to become a standard part of your clinical practice.

What the CPA hears from patients

As a chiropractor you will be rewarded daily by the opportunity you have to change people's lives for the better: 'If only I'd seen a chiropractor years ago', is a phrase the CPA hears so often.

There are many cases where patients in severe, long-term pain have turned to chiropractic as a last resort to avoid recommended, but perhaps not required, surgery.

Case study

Mrs A had suffered pain in her lower back for more years than she could remember. Nothing seemed to help except a hot water bottle for immediate relief, which she later realised, should have been a bag of frozen peas! Long walks had become increasingly painful, gardening impossible after about 15 minutes and picking up grandchildren out of the question. A friend eventually suggested consulting a chiropractor and a very sceptical Mrs A made an appointment. She was put at ease straight away by the receptionist and found the chiropractor's professional and friendly manner made her feel immediately comfortable. The first treatment brought considerable relief from pain and, after just a few more, Mrs A wrote, 'I still do have bad days but the pain has improved considerably. I already feel a different person with a very significant reduction in my pain and discomfort. I can now often sleep all night without waking up in agony'. Her chiropractor, realising Mrs A's apprehension, had opted for a gentle but effective technique, combined with addressing some of the lifestyle causes of her problem and a home muscular rehabilitation programme to prevent future episodes.

Case study

John's original back problem had started with too much rugby and road running. Over a 20-year period he had successful treatment from an osteopath and kept himself generally fit. However, he retired aged 55 and started to work for himself as a consultant. He stopped his exercise regime and spent much time travelling in cars. Eventually John had a massive spasm attack and ended up in hospital for three days, away from his local area. A combination of morphine, valium, anti-inflammatory tablets and painkillers got him back on his feet and able to travel home. He immediately went to his GP who referred him to an NHS consultant and recommended continuing the medication. John's range of movement was severely limited, and then three weeks later another bout of extreme pain led to foot drop (a paralysis or weakness in certain muscles of the foot) and a further decrease in mobility.

The appointment with the NHS consultant had still not come through, so John decided, reluctantly, to see a private orthopaedic consultant. An MRI scan revealed degeneration of the spine: at least two prolapsed discs, narrowing of channels, thinning of discs and a trapped nerve causing the foot drop. The consultant recommended an operation as soon as possible but this could not be done for six weeks and he gave no advice on management during the wait. In desperation, John's friends and family suggested he see a chiropractor. At the first appointment it was obvious that the chiropractor had a clear understanding of the MRI scan and it was agreed that he would work with John for at least the six-week period prior to surgery. A combination of treatment methods, including gentle, carefully-executed spinal manipulation, electrical stimulation and acupuncture transformed his situation and after just two weeks John turned down the surgery. His chiropractor provided an exercise programme and recommended certain activities, which he followed to the letter. After six months he was a different person: swimming, walking for up to four hours on mountain treks and embracing an active life. John is eternally grateful to his chiropractor and, especially, for the time he took to explain the plan for managing his condition and that it would not be a quick fix.

'I think one of the most important points to emphasise to others about my job is that not all my time is spent adjusting patients. Through talking to them, gaining their trust and learning about their lifestyles and activities, I am able to help improve their quality of their life and, in some cases, help them achieve their ambitions too.'

Case study

Zach developed his taste for kayaking when he was just eight years old. It took over from all his other interests in life and by the time he was 13 he was one of the sport's talented young athletes. Returning from his paper round one morning before school he suffered continuous pain in his inner pelvic region and lower back and was forced to spend the next fortnight on a sofa. His local doctor referred him to a consultant who could not solve the problem. A further series of medical tests and an MRI scan finally revealed that Zach had one leg longer than the other, his pelvis was growing too fast for his body and he would need an operation to rectify the problem. By chance, a family friend suggested visiting a local chiropractor.

The first appointment was an hour-long assessment of Zach's condition, which led to the explanation that his pain was due to a misalignment of the vertebrae in his back. He did not, in fact, have one leg longer than the other as the problem was due to a misaligned pelvis rather than an overgrown one. The misalignment in his vertebrae was putting pressure on his nerves and causing the pain. The chiropractor recommended a series of daily stretches and exercises alongside his treatment and within four weeks Zach was out of a wheelchair and able to walk. His progress continued and he recaptured his love of kayaking, which led eventually to him winning a world championship as part of the British white water rafting team and so fulfilling a decade of dreams.

Top tip

There will be times when your diagnosis of a condition and referral to another healthcare professional can avoid life-threatening complications.

Case study

An elderly lady, Mrs M, attended a chiropractor complaining of neck and upper back pain with stiffness, which had been present for some months. Her symptoms were made worse with movement and she had recently noticed a sensation of pins and needles in both arms, together with unsteadiness when walking and standing for any length of time. A thorough physical examination showed that all Mrs M's symptoms could be reproduced by various orthopaedic and neurological chiropractic tests. The chiropractor arranged for some blood tests by direct referral to Mrs M's GP and recent X-rays of her neck were made available for viewing by the local hospital. As a result, the chiropractor made a preliminary diagnosis of cervical myelopathy (an uncommon condition in which pressure was placed on the spinal cord in the neck region by degenerative bony spurs).

Mrs M's blood test results proved normal, thus ruling out any infection or other disease, and the chiropractor and GP both agreed that she should be seen with all haste by a Consultant Neurosurgeon. A fortnight later she had surgery to remove the bony spurs and widen the spinal canal. In the words of the surgeon, 'if the problem had not been realised as quickly as it was, then the consequences could have been a permanent loss of one or more neurological functions'. Mrs M recovered well from the surgery and rapidly returned to a healthy lifestyle.

BPP LEARNING MEDIA

Chapter summary

The CPA receives many stories such as the ones detailed in this chapter, in which chiropractic has changed a life. Every day you treat patients it will be a special day for at least one person, as you may be able to give them instant release from pain or hope that chronic pain and discomfort can be managed to provide a better quality of life. If you enjoy interacting with people, have patience, understanding and a keen interest in the human body, then a career helping others in this remarkable way may be right for you.

Key points

- The Chiropractic Patients' Association (CPA) is a registered charity founded by grateful patients.

- The CPA increases awareness of chiropractic and supports chiropractic research and education.

- The CoC Lay Partnership Group liaises with all other chiropractic bodies in the interests of patients.

- Chiropractors can help improve a patient's quality of life and achieve their ambitions.

- Numerous patients benefit from chiropractic care, but often seek it as a last resort.

- Sometimes your diagnosis and timely referral as a chiropractor can save a life.

Useful resources

The Chiropractic Patients' Association: www.chiropatients.org.uk

The College of Chiropractors: www.colchiro.org.uk

The General Chiropractic Council: www.gcc-uk.org

Chapter 4

How to ensure chiropractic is the right career for you

Peter Dixon

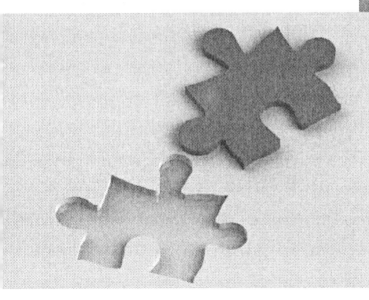

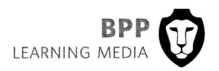

Chiropractic is the best-kept secret in healthcare. It presents the opportunity to help patients, to make a real difference to people's lives and to enter a fulfilling and rewarding profession. Deciding to become a chiropractic student will be one of the biggest decisions you will ever make, and embarking on a career in chiropractic will alter your perception of the world and provide you with great opportunities.

The profession is one of nine regulated healthcare professions in the UK, which means that it is subject to an Act of Parliament and has a professional regulatory body. There are currently around 3,000 registered chiropractors in this country, though the profession is much larger elsewhere in the world. One of the reasons the profession is relatively small in the UK is because there were no chiropractic training establishments available in the UK until 1969, and before then it was necessary to travel to the USA or Canada to train. So that leaves plenty of time and opportunity for the profession to grow!

What is the current status of the profession?

The profession in the UK is now growing, with three university-accredited undergraduate degree programmes enrolling up to 300 students per year. Acceptance of the chiropractic approach to managing neuro-musculoskeletal disorders related to the spine and other joints is gaining increasing acceptance. Like any healthcare discipline, chiropractic combines a science-based training with the need to have an empathy with patients and finding satisfaction in helping them. The basic pre-clinical science training is similar to that in a medical school and, as a result, some subjects required for entry are similar.

Top tip

There are currently only three places to train in the UK so there is competition for places, which tends to put upward pressure on the entry requirements.

If you are able to study full-time, the shortest training programme is four years, but longer programmes are available if you are returning to work or cannot manage week-on-week commitments. Either way, the training will need your strong commitment, but the rewards of being a chiropractor at the end will be worth the effort.

What do you want from your career?

You need to think carefully about what you want from any career before you commit to it. Education now involves considerable resources, so it is wise to take care when considering your options, see Chapter 7. First, you need to understand what being a chiropractor means and what it entails, and then you should to ask yourself what you want to be doing in five, ten or 15 years time.

> **Top tip**
>
> Whether chiropractic is your first career, or if you are changing career, you have to be able to visualise yourself in your new professional role.

If you are going to embrace a career, then it is much easier if it is going to be something you enjoy. If you enjoy meeting a wide variety of people, are happy with building relationships quickly and are able to make decisions with confidence, then you may well be suited to being a chiropractor. But if you find it hard to meet and engage with people on a one-to-one basis, then you may struggle. Basically, you need to like people to consider chiropractic in the first instance.

The training is science-based so you should ideally have an interest in science. As an independent practitioner you need to be able to analyse a situation, make decisions and act upon them, but you do not need to be an academic genius to qualify. The programmes are pretty rigorous, however, as you will be responsible ultimately for the patient under your personal care, so you will need to be dedicated to studying and completing the course workload.

> **Top tip**
>
> Consider contacting a local chiropractor and asking to sit in and observe them at work. They may be able to suggest other colleagues that would be happy to talk to you. You should also aim to be adjusted yourself, if you are not already under chiropractic care, so that you can start to understand what it might feel like for a patient. The more you can learn about the profession before you decide to start training, the better.

What motivates you?

While it is possible to make a good living from a career in chiropractor, if money is your main motivation then perhaps another job may be more suitable. If job satisfaction is important to you, however, then chiropractic offers that in abundance. It is a great privilege to be able to help someone improve their health. Chiropractic is an excellent example of *piece work*: there is a cost per session and your earnings are directly related to the number of patients you see. As you develop your practice there may be other business opportunities that you can develop but, basically, the more patients you see, the more you earn.

Top tip

The kind of piece work that chiropractic offers means that you can decide to work when you like and as much as you like. This often suits people who are making lifestyle choices and want some flexibility in their working life.

What are the key practice choices?

The technical aspects of the treatment will be explained elsewhere (see Chapter 11), but there are distinct elements of the job that are worth initial exploration. While the scope of chiropractic practice can be as wide as you choose, it is essentially restricted to either clinical practice or research / academia, although chiropractors also get involved in teaching and in the regulatory elements of the profession. A career in medicine presents a doctor with a multitude of clinical disciplines and environments, but a clinical chiropractic career is usually undertaken in a private clinic environment. There are some opportunities for working within a General Practitioner's (GP's) practice or in a hospital, but these tend to be as an independent clinician rather than as part of an extended team. Your main clinical chiropractic career option will be as a sole practitioner in a consulting room within a private practice, and this requires an ability to make diagnostic decisions and implement them without immediate reference to other people. This scenario may change, however, as the profession becomes more integrated into the healthcare system.

Case study: Newly-qualified chiropractor

'Some time ago I came across some professional people who really cared about my welfare, not only physically but mentally – they were chiropractors. They helped me immensely with the pain I was experiencing but also made sense of what had happened to me and how it was affecting my body and mind. I will always be grateful for their understanding, caring and compassionate ways and they inspired me to start this journey to become a chiropractor.

From Year 1 the subjects were hard, but interesting at the same time. Realising that there was a complete new language called 'medical terminology', and being able to understand it, was at times frustrating; finding out that every nook, cranny and bump of the body had an individual name was overwhelming at times; and having to learn chemistry and biomechanics for the first time was a challenge. Well done to those tutors who had the hard task of teaching me these subjects and making them understandable. All of my hard work paid off though in the final clinic year, when I was able to treat patients who needed my help and everything really started to come to come together.

This programme helped me to believe in myself and really boosted my self-confidence. During the years there were many ups and downs and it has taken a lot of perseverance and determination to get here, but now it is done I can finally do what I have wanted to do for so long – help people just as I was helped myself.'

Independent practice

Private practice is a uniquely challenging and satisfying experience. You have to establish and build your business in the first instance, of course, but then how you practise is up to you. If you join an established practice you will need to develop your own patient base within that practice, but you will get help and support from those around you as you take those first steps into practice life. You could also set up practice for yourself: by hiring a room in a sports clinic, a complementary health clinic or a GP's surgery. Either way, you will be an independent practitioner regardless of your employment circumstances and will need to be registered with the General Chiropractic Council (GCC) in order to practise in the UK.

'There are some major advantages of being a registered healthcare professional: acceptance by the medical profession and the confidence that registration instils in patients, plus the fact that all the private medical insurance companies now recognise chiropractic for reimbursement.'

Do you have the right qualities for chiropractic?

Do you want to help people, do you have good communication skills and can you make decisions under pressure? These are all necessary skills for a chiropractic career. You might not be sure at the moment whether you have the skills, but if you have the right motivation and commitment then the chiropractic programme will provide you with the necessary knowledge to support your decisions and help you to develop your communication skills.

Top tip

It is a good idea to consider discussing your career choice with family and friends to see what they think, as they will probably know you pretty well and may give you the confidence you need to decide to take the next step.

Chiropractic feels right for you, so what next?

Before committing yourself to a programme of study, you need to find out as much as you can about being a chiropractic student as well as a chiropractor (see Chapter 9). The best way to do this is to talk to as many people as possible. There is no substitute for experience, so take the time to visit one or more of the colleges. Try to attend the open days that they hold and take every opportunity to observe chiropractors at work.

Consider in advance what you will need to gain a place at one of the colleges (see Chapter 5). All potential candidates will need the necessary academic qualifications, but what will make you stand out from the crowd? If there is competition for places, the decision about awarding places may well rest on the non-academic, extra-curricular, aspects of your application. These will fall broadly into the following categories:

*   Communication skills
*   Work experience in a chiropractic clinic

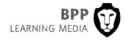

- Teamwork and leadership promise
- Likely contribution to student life
- Family, friends (and you!) receiving chiropractic care
- Experience in other aspects of your life
- Self-reliance and sense of responsibility
- Potential for developing the profession

Taking each aspect in turn, think about your relevant skills and experience in each category and how they might impact on your training and, eventually, on your work as a chiropractor. Think about whether you can do something now that will boost your application in the future. There is no standard that you must achieve in each category, but every extra tick in the box can make a difference to the total picture.

Communication skills

As with any job that involves dealing with people, communication is vital. You need to be able to engage with your patients and the faster you can develop a rapport, the more successful you will be. As a student this is very important as well. You will be part of a year group, and if relationships within that group are harmonious and supportive, then all members of the group will be more successful. Often your student year group will become your friends for life. Part of the entry process will be an interview and you need to be able to demonstrate your communication skills then but, more importantly, you need to understand the importance of such skills and try to develop and improve them in order to enhance your chances of success throughout your career.

Top tip

Remember, as a chiropractor, you will have to explain to patients what their problem may be and what you are going to do about it. The better you communicate with them, the more confidence they will have in you.

Work experience

Work experience is invaluable, even if it is only observational, and the more practices you visit, the better equipped you will be to start training and then enter practice after graduation. When you visit a practice, try to understand all aspects of work there, and also take notes. These will be valuable as evidence of your enquiries and they will also help you in formulating your thoughts about chiropractic as a career. If you have

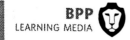

BPP
LEARNING MEDIA

pursued other activities, at school and after school, such as community-based work or anything that demonstrates a caring and supportive role, it will be helpful. Other experiences, such as travelling, can add to a college application, especially if you can demonstrate that what you have learnt while travelling has helped you in making your decision to become a chiropractor.

Leadership and responsibility

Any opportunity that you have to demonstrate your leadership skills and your ability to take on responsibility will help you in your application to train, and also in your work as a chiropractor. In practice, your patients will be looking to you for a lead both in the treatment you provide and the advice that you give. You will have a very high level of responsibility as a chiropractor in that you will be a primary contact practitioner – you are not relying on a previous health screen before referral. When you graduate and enter the profession, you will find yourself in a leadership role in which you may have clinic staff that require managing. There will be a gradual progression towards this, but leadership is a key skill if you are to be successful.

Teamwork

While a lot of the work of a chiropractor is one-to-one with the patient, you will still be part of a team. As a student you will be required to enter into joint learning activities, especially in the technique classes, and later you will need to understand how to build a team with your colleagues within your practice and other colleagues locally. Successful relationships make for successful practices, and as a private practitioner this is extremely important.

Contribution to student life

Well-rounded, sociable people will contribute positively to the student experience for everyone and will ultimately make good chiropractors. This is what the colleges are hoping to produce, so if you can demonstrate your abilities in these fields you will be a more attractive proposition as a student and a greater success as a chiropractor.

'I have never met a chiropractor who did not enjoy their practice every single day. I am not sure there are many professions that can say that.'

Chapter summary

Chiropractic presents a unique way of looking at health and a different way of handling the needs of patients. It is not a 'mainstream' healthcare profession, although great strides have been made to make chiropractic available within this context. It is, however, a profession that is accepted within the modern healthcare system in the UK and that provides many avenues for professional growth. When you apply, you will be starting on a journey that will provide you with a professional, caring and rewarding profession.

Key points

- Chiropractic is one of nine regulated healthcare professions in the UK.
- There are three university-accredited undergraduate degree programmes to consider.
- Before applying, understand what being a chiropractor means and what it entails.
- Consider your motives: life plan; money; job satisfaction.
- Review the necessary skills you will need for a chiropractic career.
- Visit the colleges, observe other chiropractors and ask questions.

Useful resources

Chiropractors Act 1994:
www.legislation.gov.uk/ukpga/1994/17/contents

The General Chiropractic Council: www.gcc-uk.org

BPP LEARNING MEDIA

Chapter 5

What is involved in the application process?

Gayle Hoffman and Jane Cooke

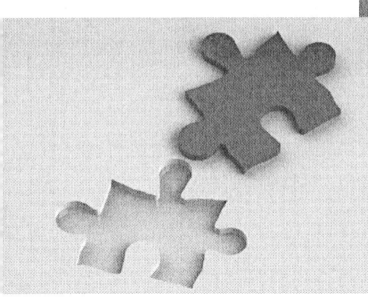

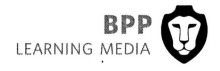

BPP
LEARNING MEDIA

Congratulations, if you have decided that chiropractic is the career for you! In this chapter you will find out what you need to do in order to apply to study at one of the three institutions currently conferring a chiropractic qualification in the UK. Your application will normally involve a UCAS (Universities and Colleges Admissions Service) application form, a college application form and an interview. A key consideration may be where you live and whether you are prepared to, or can afford to, relocate for your studies. Fortunately, there are some options for distance learning, so you do not necessarily have to 'uproot' to pursue this career.

Fee structures vary between colleges and there are some favourable student loans and bursaries / scholarships available, all of which you will need to consider (see Chapter 7). If you are concerned that your secondary education qualifications may not make you eligible to apply, there are foundation programmes on offer for those without A levels in science or vocational qualifications in a hands-on therapy.

Pre-chiropractic access programmes

Pre-chiropractic foundation programmes, sometimes called pathway or access programmes, are an option for candidates who do not have the required basic science A level subjects for immediate degree entry, but who have demonstrated academic ability or qualifications in another field. These programmes run for an academic year and are available at all the colleges. Some, like the McTimoney College pathway programme (the Pathway to HE Certificate in Health) are essentially open access as long as you can demonstrate your commitment to complete the programme, while others like the Welsh Institute of Chiropractic programme require 240 UCAS points for entry to their foundation year programme. The Anglo European College of Chiropractic runs an Access to Higher Education Diploma (Human Health Sciences), for those seeking access to health related higher education degrees, such as chiropractic. (See Chapter 6.) All three colleges are located south of Oxford, but the McTimoney College Pathway programme will also be run from central Manchester from January 2013.

The UCAS form

Applications for acceptance on to one of the chiropractic colleges are initially made through UCAS, although you can contact any of the colleges directly to begin with if you wish. There are three colleges in the UK that currently offer a master's degree in chiropractic:

- Anglo-European College of Chiropractic (AECC, Bournemouth)
- McTimoney College of Chiropractic (MCC, Oxfordshire)
- Welsh Institute of Chiropractic (WIOC, Glamorgan)

These colleges have university validation, which means that they have recognised tertiary education status in the UK, and they are recognised by the General Chiropractic Council (GCC), as follows: the Anglo-European College of Chiropractic (AECC), validated by Bournemouth University, the McTimoney College of Chiropractic (MCC), validated by BBP University College, and the Welsh Institute of Chiropractic (WIOC) validated by the University of Glamorgan.

The general entry requirement for a chiropractic master's programme is the completion of three A levels, including sciences (preferably Biology, Chemistry or Physics). The number of UCAS points required for entry to the master's degree varies between the colleges: at the time of writing, AECC requires 280, MCC requires 260 and WIOC requires 320 UCAS points (with 240 for the foundation programme). Whatever your level of academic achievement, it is important to know that a significant part of the UCAS form (which you have control over) is your personal statement. This helps the admissions office choose those applicants who will be shortlisted.

Top tip

There may be some programmes that require you to apply directly to the college concerned. If you do not see the programme you are interested in on the UCAS site, phone the college directly and ask them for details of any specific procedures that you need to follow.

The personal statement

Your UCAS personal statement is your chance to be creative and think of yourself as a young 'Di Vinci' with a blank canvas and new brushes to explain why you should be offered a place over your rivals applying for the same programme. Please remember that you can only write one personal statement and that statement will be used for all your applications.

Chiropractic colleges are looking for individuals who will have the necessary qualities and attributes to become their professional colleagues on graduation. Chiropractic is a regulated health profession and, in practice, you will need to demonstrate the highest standards of professional and personal conduct. For that reason the colleges will

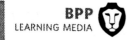

be looking, not only at your qualifications, but also at why you want to become a chiropractor. For example, have you, or your family, been helped by chiropractic and as a result do you want to help others? Or have you been inspired by a local chiropractor by watching them in practice? Importantly, they will be looking to see whether you have the commitment and enthusiasm to complete the programme.

The average ratio of applicants to college places is about three to one, so you will need to stand out from other applicants in order to be accepted. The personal statement is your first opportunity to do this.

Writing your UCAS personal statement

- Make your introduction attention grabbing: keep in mind that you will need to stand out and that a great introduction will encourage further reading.

- Show your enthusiasm by demonstrating an insight into your chosen profession, along with your commitment to the field.

- Have you been to observe a chiropractor or are you and your family under chiropractic care?

- Ask yourself, 'What qualities do I have to make myself suitable for the profession?'

- Incorporate your academic and extra-curricular activities into your admission statement.

- Double check, 'Is the information I am providing relevant for the programmes that I am applying for?'

- Ensure that all information you give is accurate information as this is the stepping stone for your interview and you may be asked to expand further.

- Check your statement for spelling and grammar mistakes and stay within the guidelines of the word limit.

- Make sure your personal statement contains a short concluding paragraph: a strong closure may stay in the forefront of interviewers' minds and help put you on the shortlist for the next phase of your application process.

Top tip

UCAS provides an online personal statement worksheet that you can use to put down your thoughts and help you through the process of writing down your personal statement.

The General Chiropractic Council's Equality and Diversity Scheme

In May 2009, the GCC reviewed and updated its Equality and Diversity Scheme. It is an example of the profession's commitment to the promotion and protection of equality and diversity within the chiropractic profession, as well as within the council's own workforce. The GCC also has a *Guide for Disabled Students* (2010). See Useful resources.

The interview

You will be required to attend an interview prior to a college making you an offer. Once you get to this stage, congratulate yourself as it shows you have done extremely well and that the admissions team have seen something promising in your application. Now you will need to begin the preparation for your interview. The interview process is an opportunity to assess your motivation, commitment and your ability to adapt to the rigours of the chiropractic programme. There may be two or three interviewers present and your interview will last for anything between ten to 30 minutes, so stay calm and show your best qualities!

*'For me the interview is an opportunity to listen to the student's individual story. Most of all, I am interested in **why** they want to become a chiropractor because they will need motivation and commitment in order to complete the programme.'* **Member of college admissions staff**

Some colleges may ask you to attend an open day prior to interview. It may be that you can have an interview on the same day as the open day. This provides a very good opportunity to have a look around and speak to some of the staff and it also allows you to settle and feel less nervous before the actual interview itself. Do try to present yourself at your best. You must feel comfortable in your interview clothes, but above all you will need to dress smartly and professionally to give your interviewers a good impression of the chiropractor you intend to be.

Application and interview advice

Most college application forms and interview questions are meant to help you and the college find out if the programme is a good match for you. You will rarely get a question that 'puts you on the spot' or makes you feel inadequate in any way. Remember, the college is trying to make a good impression too. Use the interview to show off your personality in ways that are not possible on an application form. Below are some typical interview questions and some suggestions for answering them:

'Tell us about yourself'

This question seems easier than it is. How do you reduce your whole life to a few sentences? Try to say something memorable that really makes you different from other college applicants.

'Why are you interested in our college?'

Be specific when answering this, and show that you have done your research. What is it about the college that distinguishes it from other establishments that you are considering?

'What can we tell you about our college?'

It is highly likely that your interviewer will provide an opportunity for you to ask questions. Make sure you have some, and that your questions are thoughtful and specific to the particular college. Think of some probing and focused questions, for example, 'What would graduates of your college consider to be the most valuable aspect of their time spent here?'

'Do you have any special interests?'

You do not need to have decided upon a specialist type of practice when you apply to chiropractic college. However, if you are interested in a particular field of practice (working with animals or children, for example), come prepared to explain why.

'What will you contribute to our student community?'

You will want to be specific when answering this question. Think about what it is that makes 'you' uniquely 'you', and what exactly will you bring to diversify the college community.

'Tell us about a challenge that you overcame.'

This question is designed to see what kind of problem-solver you are. When confronted with a challenge, how do you handle the situation? College will be full of challenges and problem-solving is an essential attribute for a chiropractor.

'What are your hobbies?'

College life is not all work and no play, so the admissions staff may favour students who pursue interesting and productive hobbies at leisure. Do you write? Are you well read? Do you practise a sport? Use a question such as this one to show that you are well-rounded with a variety of interests.

'Can you give me an example of when you have worked in a team?'

Teamwork is an essential part of healthcare practice, either with other chiropractors or health professionals in the community. There will be many ways that you can show that you are a team player, such as being part of a sports team, sitting on a committee or organising an event. You might also be able to illustrate leadership skills through teamwork, whether as the captain of your sports team or simply examples where you have made a decision that has led to others taking a different direction and following your lead.

'Where do you see yourself in five to ten years time?'

You do not need to pretend that you have your future worked out if you get a question like this. Very few students entering college can accurately predict their future. However, your interviewer does want to see that you think ahead. If you can see yourself doing, say, three specific things in the future, express yourself. Honesty and open-mindedness will work in your favour.

'Does your school or career record reflect your effort and ability?'

In the interview or on your application form, you often have an opportunity to explain a bad grade or misguided career choice. Take care here – you do not want to come across as a whiner or as someone who blames others for a problem. However, if you have had extenuating circumstances, let the college know.

'If you could change one thing in your past, what would it be?'

A question like this can turn sour if you make the mistake of dwelling on things you regret, so stay positive. Perhaps you have always wondered if you would have enjoyed a career in acting or music. Maybe, in retrospect, studying massage might have been more in line with your career goals than studying French. A good answer may show that you have not yet had enough time to explore everything that interests you.

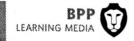

Case study: Second year student

'Going through the UCAS application process isn't complex. It gave me the chance to show off my skills, qualifications and experiences in a personal statement and provided a useful space to explain why I wanted to study chiropractic at which particular college. UCAS is also good as you can track the status of your application instantly online and do not have to rely on the postman!

I recommend attending an open day before submitting your application. It tells you what the course is all about, but also allows you to ask questions and meet some of the tutors and staff before you start. Attending an open day is rewarding as you can meet other people and gain their perspectives on why they are passionate about studying chiropractic.

I don't know anyone who is fond of interviews, but my interview was far from scary – it was more like a friendly, informal chat. I felt the interviewer drew the best out of me and did not try to trip me up. Most particularly, I found the interview helpful in establishing and clarifying anything I had not considered before starting the course.'

Chapter summary

You will only get one chance to fill in your UCAS form each academic year, so think ahead to all the colleges you are applying to. You can improve your submission if you have thoroughly researched all your target institutions and if you make a strong and personal case for enrolment. Remember, you can use the UCAS website for help, and always ask someone to proofread your form before you submit it. Your college interview may be the first one you have had, so be prepared. The more you can rehearse, the brighter you will shine on the day of the interview. Practice will also help you identify habits that you may have without realising – not making eye contact, for example. On the day of the interview, remember to arrive on time and dress professionally... and good luck. If you are bright, diligent, patient and caring this profession needs you!

Key points

- In order to eventually practise as a chiropractor, you must have the minimum of a degree validated by a UK-recognised higher education institution.

- You must adhere to the UCAS deadlines.

- Make your personal statement concise, reflective and relevant to chiropractic.

- The key to a great interview is preparation and practice beforehand.

Useful resources

BBP University College: www.bbp.com

Bournemouth University: www.bournemouth.ac.uk

GCC equality and diversity scheme:

Open University: www.open-university.co.uk

UCAS: www.ucas.ac.uk

University of Glamorgan: www.glam.ac.uk

www.gcc-uk.org/files/link_file/Agreed_Equality_and_Diversity_
Scheme_May_09_FINAL.pdf

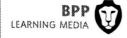

Chapter 6

How do I choose which programme to apply for?

Jane Cooke

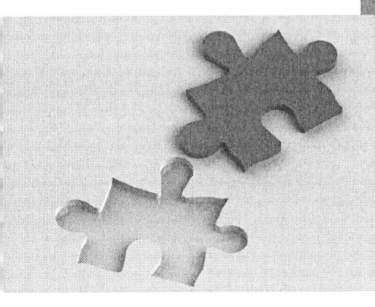

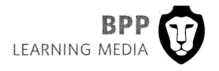

When considering where to apply, there are currently only three chiropractic colleges to choose from, so your pre-college research will not be complicated compared with other UK primary healthcare career choices. However, there has been some interest in starting new colleges / programmes, so is always worth checking the education pages of the General Chiropractic Council (GCC) website in case other programmes are available in the future. The three colleges are the Anglo European College of Chiropractic (AECC), the McTimoney College of Chiropractic (MCC) and the Welsh Institute of Chiropractic (WIOC), all of which have university accreditation, offer master's level programmes, and are recognised by the General Chiropractic Council, the regulatory body for chiropractic in the UK. (See also Chapter 5.) All the programmes meet the published criteria for degree recognition, but each of them has their own ideology and approach. You can only register and practise as a chiropractor in the UK if you have graduated from one of these programmes. In this chapter, you can find out·more about the individual colleges and what they have to offer, and also get a taste of which appeals most to your personal philosophy and perspective.

The Anglo-European College of Chiropractic

The AECC is in Bournemouth on the south coast, a location with good road and rail access and a local airport with connections to mainland Europe. The AECC is an independent Higher Education Institution and is associated with Bournemouth University. The main programme provided by the college is the BSc / MSc Chiropractic, which is a five-year full-time chiropractic programme. To graduate as a chiropractor from the AECC on this programme you are required to complete the full-time three-year BSc (Hons) Human Sciences degree followed by the full-time two-year postgraduate MSc Chiropractic degree.

The BSc segment of the programme covers anatomy, physiology, biochemistry, biomechanics, and chiropractic skills (see Chapters 10 and 11), including contact with patients and clinical case studies from the outset. Students completing these three years successfully, in addition to the Clinic Entrance Qualifying Examination, progress to the MSc qualification. The MSc level is largely based on clinical internship, which students undertake in the AECC student clinic, treating patients in a supervised environment.

The BSc / MSc Chiropractic is an integrated programme of study and is designed to train and prepare students for professional practice as primary healthcare providers in modern society. It gives students real-life experience as they are exposed to clinical case studies and patients from the start. The AECC has been established for over 50 years and prides itself on its ability and eagerness to be at the forefront of musculoskeletal research and innovation.

Other AECC programmes

In addition to the BSc / MSc Chiropractic programme, the AECC offers, together with Bournemouth University, a BSc (Hons) Exercise Science (Health and Rehabilitation) degree programme, accredited by the British Association of Sports and Exercise Science (BASES). This programme is intended to provide students with a foundation for safe and competent practice in the area of exercise programme design and implementation. It also opens up a range of opportunities for careers in healthcare and / or further studies in health-related disciplines. Another programme offered by the AECC is the BSc (Hons) Community Health and Rehabilitation, a flexible three-year programme oriented toward community health and rehabilitation, which is targeted at school leavers, career change individuals and healthcare professionals who want to develop or add to their skills and knowledge of community health.

A further range of MSc programmes in Diagnostic Ultrasound and Advanced Professional Practice are also available, and these include clinical sciences, paediatric musculoskeletal health, musculoskeletal rehabilitation, sports and rehabilitation, and orthopaedics. The AECC's Access to Higher Education Diploma (Human Health Sciences) programme is designed for those seeking access to health-related higher education programmes or degrees, such as chiropractic, exercise science, community health and rehabilitation, physiotherapy, osteopathy or other health sciences. This programme is part-time and covers the range of skills required to progress to further study once completed.

AECC key benefits

- It is the oldest college in the UK attracting students from all over the world.

- The College achieves high levels of student satisfaction.

- Over 50% of students come from outside the UK, creating a vibrant, multicultural place to study.

- Students get extensive hands-on clinical experience from the start.

- Facilities include purpose-built teaching clinics, with high-tech functional exercise and rehabilitation centre, diagnostic ultrasound, X-ray and fluoroscopy facilities.

- There are excellent campus facilities, including extensive library and learning resources, cafeteria and sports hall.

- College research and clinical expertise are recognised globally.

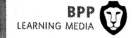

AECC application codes

The associated UCAS course codes for the BSc / MSc in Chiropractic are as follows (for details of the other course codes, please visit the college website):

Institution code name: AECC
Institution code: A65
Course code: B321

Top tip

Open days

All three colleges offer regular open or visitor days and these should be an essential part of your college research. They allow you to explore the campuses and facilities, ask staff questions and meet current students and potential applicants like yourself. Visit the college websites or call the admissions offices to find out about dates.

The McTimoney College of Chiropractic

The MCC is located in Abingdon, just south of Oxford. It is a short drive from the A34 and within easy access of the M4 and M40. The nearest train stations are Didcot Parkway and Oxford. The MCC offers a range of study programmes at foundation, undergraduate and postgraduate levels. The Integrated Master's in Chiropractic (MChiro) is the key route for registration with the GCC and a career in chiropractic. The college offers a standard full-time and a unique full-time extended delivery option so that you can continue to work in your pre-clinical years of study.

At the MCC there are two routes to the master's degree: a four-year pathway, which follows a standard academic year with studies delivered during the week. Three years of academic and practical studies (around 20 hours a week) are followed by a full-time clinical year treating patients under supervision in the college's community clinic. The five-year extended pathway, which commences each January, is the only programme which offers students the possibility of studying at weekends and in summer schools. This means that you can still continue to work if you wish alongside your studies. If you choose this option, four years of academic and practical studies delivered on campus and through directed studies are followed by a full-time clinical year. The college also offers a foundation programme, the Pathway to HE Certificate in Health, which has been designed specifically for those wishing to join a chiropractic programme but who do not have the required UCAS points for A level passes or equivalent. From January 2013 this will be delivered in Abingdon and also central Manchester.

> *'I always wanted to help others in any way I could so I set out to achieve my dream. I enrolled on the access course and then successfully continued on to the chiropractic programme. I couldn't have done it any other way.'* **Chiropractic student**

Postgraduate MSc programmes

The MCC is the only college in the world to offer externally validated master's-level programmes that enable successful graduates to use chiropractic techniques on animals. You must already have a recognised degree in chiropractic, osteopathy or physiotherapy in order to gain direct entry to the two-year MSc Animal Manipulation, which trains you to care for horses, dogs and farm animals. If you are not already a qualified registered practitioner but have science-based animal qualifications, for example, equine science or zoology degrees, you will first need to undertake the Animal Foundation Programme supplied by the College. If you are a trained osteopath, you can choose the MSc Animal Manipulation (Osteopathic Pathway), also a two-year programme, and the only master's programme in Europe that trains students in animal osteopathic techniques (See Chapter 14).

Case study: New animal master's graduate

'I originally heard about chiropractic from the animal side of things and was amazed after seeing the benefits that the treatment had on both my horse and my dog. My horse suddenly became reluctant to be ridden and seemed fretful. Our vet was busy but an animal chiropractor was visiting another horse in our stables. She volunteered to check him and found a hoof abscess that needed to be treated by the vet. However, as I learned that my horse had been compensating for the infection for some time, the chiropractor returned to rectify the muscular imbalances that had been caused. With my dog, it was incredible! She had been hit by a car several years ago and couldn't run or jump like other dogs – we just came to accept this. The same chiropractor made some adjustments to her lower spine and straight after the treatment she was leaping up at me, just like a puppy.

I signed up for the chiropractic programme and have now just completed my animal master's as well, so I am properly qualified in both disciplines. The years have flown by and I have loved all of it, apart from the revising!'

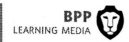

The MSc Chiropractic (Small Animals) is a one-year programme that prepares the student to care for dogs, cats and other small pets, and is only open to qualified chiropractors. The MCC also offers a practice-based MSc Chiropractic (Paediatrics) programme for qualified chiropractors, which takes three years to complete.

Established for 40 years, the College emphasises training in the McTimoney method of chiropractic, which is a gentle and holistic treatment developed by founder John McTimoney who began teaching his methods in 1972. As the smallest College it creates a friendly and supportive learning environment especially for mature students. There is a very good ratio of tutors to students, especially in the practical training modules, and it has a strong research culture with a good track record of publishing student projects. In addition to the academic modules and clinical training provided by all chiropractic degree programmes, the MCC places a strong emphasis on teaching the philosophy of chiropractic.

MCC key benefits

- The College offers unique extended study programmes to fit in with your other commitments so you can study while you continue to work.

- The McTimoney method of chiropractic is taught only at the MCC and is highly sought after by patients.

- The College provides a supportive, professional and student-focused study environment.

- The master's degree programmes include animal manipulation available only at the MCC.

- MCC has a strong involvement in chiropractic research with many important and current academic papers published by staff and students.

- There are custom-designed, state-of-the-art rooms and facilities including an on-site chiropractic clinic.

- There is a vibrant student community with opportunities to take part in international student events linked to the College's worldwide contacts.

MCC application codes

Chiropractic programmes at the university and the associated UCAS course codes for the Integrated Master's in Chiropractic (MChiro) are as follows (for details of the other course codes, please visit the College website):

- Institution code name: BPP
  Institution code: B54
  Campus code: A

- Four-year programme course code: B320

- Five-year programme course code: BH20

The Welsh Institute of Chiropractic

WIOC is in Pontypridd near Cardiff, Wales. It is close to junction 32 of the M4 and there is a train station nearby (Treforest Station). The programme is a four-year, full-time Integrated Master of Chiropactic (MChiro) degree run according to a standard academic year. Typically, you will spend around 20–24 hours each week in lectures, practical sessions, laboratory and clinical work. The modules you will cover are similar to those offered on all the chiropractic degree programmes and will include basic human sciences, clinical training, practising in a student clinic and a research project (see Chapters 10, 11 and 16). WIOC also offers a Pre-Chiropractic Foundation Year programme for those without the required UCAS points for A level passes or equivalent for prospective students wanting to pursue a health professional career who have no science background. The Foundation Year aims to prepare students for the rigours of the MChiro programme and students must attain an overall 60% average in all modules to progress to the degree.

The WIOC chiropractic degree will enable you to develop a critical, analytical and evaluative approach to the principles and practice of chiropractic. You will gain investigative skills and see chiropractic in the context of all other health-related professions. Your chiropractic training means you will understand the scientific principles relevant to chiropractic, and be able to diagnose and manage a range of relevant, health-related conditions. To improve your employability, this degree includes practical skills relevant to professional practice and effective communication skills, as well as an understanding of the legal and business framework of the professional chiropractor.

Other WIOC programmes

A range of sports-related degrees are delivered by the Faculty of Health, Sport and Science, and MSc programmes in Sport, Health and Exercise Science, and Performance Coaching are also available.

WIOC key benefits

- The Institute is part of a large university which enhances the overall student experience.

- There is an on-site multi-room chiropractic training clinic, X-ray and rehabilitation suites and MRI facilities.

- The Institute offers a clinical placement programme with the Local NHS Health Board.

- Student association membership is available, including conferences and involvement in promotional activities and student involvement in university sports teams, local rugby clubs and professional organisations.

- The Chiropractic Society is supported by the University of Glamorgan Students' Union.

- There is a strong emphasis on research undergraduate training and active participation in chiropractic research.

- The Institute has international links with chiropractic institutions around the world and internationally recognised members of academic staff.

WIOC application codes

The University of Glamorgan's code name is GLAM and its institution code is G14. Chiropractic programmes at the university and the associated UCAS course codes are as follows:

- MChiro Chiropractic UCAS code: B320

- Foundation Certificate Chiropractic UCAS code: B326

Chapter summary

The final choice for where you study to be a chiropractor is limited to three establishments at present and each college offers the essential master's degree in chiropractic, but there are many other factors to consider: location, budget and your own personal reasons for seeking to pursue this innovative and important career are just some examples. Do explore the options carefully – although places are limited, an early and earnest application will be positively received from each of the colleges. Open day visits and, if possible, chiropractic observations or appointments with graduates of each of the colleges will prove invaluable when considering your choice of college.

Key points

- There are currently three chiropractic colleges to choose from, all of which have university validation and are recognised by the GCC.

- You can only register and practise as a chiropractor in the UK if you have graduated from one of these colleges.

- Each college offers more than the essential master's degree in chiropractic, so do explore all the possibilities.

- Access programmes are offered by all the colleges if you do not have the pre-requisite academic requirements: typically three A levels (preferably in science).

- Open days, or visitor days, are run regularly by the colleges and are extremely worthwhile.

- Speak to a graduate or a current student of one of the colleges to gain first-hand information.

- Admissions staff will be very happy to receive a phone call or an email regarding any queries.

Useful resources

Anglo-European College of Chiropractic: www.aecc.ac.uk

General Chiropractic Council education page:
www.gcc-uk.org/page.cfm?page_id=25

McTimoney College of Chiropractic: www.mctimoney-college.ac.uk

Welsh Institute of Chiropractic: www.glam.ac.uk

Chapter 7

Student and early career finances

Michael B Bennett and
Christina Cunliffe

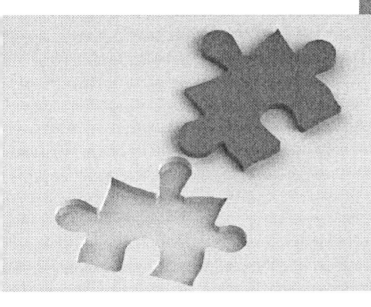

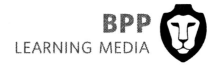

This chapter will look at the different methods of funding your chiropractic studies and also some considerations for the early years of your professional career. All degree programmes in the UK charge significant fees these days, and chiropractic training is no different in that regard. One thing to take into account, though, is that you will have a ready-made career at the end.

What you must to do though is consider carefully how much your studies will cost, and how you will fund them. You will find out very quickly that being a chiropractor is not only a career, but also a business and no matter how much you want to help people, you must think of it that way. You therefore also need to consider what your costs will be after you have graduated. This will not only take into account the repayment of any student loans you have taken out, but also the cost of registration and other professional fees, as well as the cost of running the business itself.

While finance may seem like a very intimidating subject, the good news is that there are plenty of people and organisations available to help you and we will look at some of these later on in the chapter.

The cost of training

Before embarking on a four- or five-year training course, you need to consider how much it is going to cost you (or somebody else!). From September 2012, students will have to pay £9,000 per year (nearly £12,000 if you are self-funded) and nearly £12,000 per annum for the final two years at the Anglo-European College of Chiropractic (AECC). Fees at the McTimoney College of Chiropractic (MCC) are currently £6,000 per year and £8,000 for the final clinic year. At the Welsh Institute of Chiropractic (WIOC) your fees will be £3,465 per year if you are a student from Wales and £9,000 per year if you are from England.

The cost of becoming a chiropractor can therefore range from £26,000 to just over £50,000 (or £59,000 for a self-funded student) in England. For students in Wales, the cost is just under £14,000. If you need to complete a foundation year, this can cost you an additional £1,500 in England or £3,465 in Wales.

Additional costs

You will need to buy your own text books, clinic tunics and clinical equipment. Do not underestimate how this will all add up as medical textbooks can be quite expensive. Consider whether or not you need to buy a book or use the reference books in the library – second-hand books can also be a cost-effective option (see Chapter 9). You will need to buy clinical equipment, such as a stethoscope, and it is best to choose good-quality items that will last you throughout your career.

Take advice from your lecturers and tutors before purchasing any books or equipment as they are in the best place to guide you towards the things you really need.

In some cases there are also some additional one-off registration fees and ancillary costs, such as a Criminal Record Bureau check.

Loans and funding

Most prospective students should be entitled to standard loans from Student Finance England (SFE) or Student Finance Wales (SFW). The most notable exception is if you already hold a degree. As a minimum you should be entitled to receive a student loan to cover the basic course fees up to £9,000 per year (or £6,000 for private universities). Dependent upon your household income, there may also be additional loans or grants available. As a general guide, these are readily available where your household income is £20,000 or below. There is a degree of support for households earning £20,000–£42,000, but above that level there is nothing further available.

Some banks, notably NatWest, RBS and Barclays have in the past been interested in lending money to assist students with their studies as they know that once qualified, they are likely to become a good and valued customer. These days, however, loans are more difficult to obtain generally, so you should start the process early if this is the route you need to follow.

Other funding sources

There are other ways in which programmes may be funded. The lowest cost method is invariably the 'MAD' bank; this is the bank where you never make deposits, regularly make withdrawals and never have to repay the loan. MAD stands for 'Mum And Dad' and those of you fortunate to have supportive parents may be able to avoid taking on too much student loan debt.

Case study: Final-year chiropractic student

'Lots of people leave college with student loans, but in my case I am indebted to my mum and dad whose support and belief in me was unconditional and plentiful. My wife also supported me by ironing my clinic tunics every week and put up with my grumpy and stressful moods. And they never, ever complained. I was very lucky because I lived close to the college of my choice and I didn't face travel and accommodation expenses, which can really rack up. My family did get some returns as I would treat all their aches and pains during my training, and I still provide free treatments for my family and all their friends. I am also their first port of call if they are unsure about whether they need to visit a GP or not.'

Alternatively, there is the possibility of a relative, partner or close friend who is already trading in an allied professional area and who is prepared to employ you and pay for your training (a route that is often overlooked). The costs of an employer training staff, even if it is in totally new areas of expertise, are generally allowable for tax. So if your mother is, say, a private physiotherapist, she could employ you and then pay your course fees, thus reducing her taxable profit.

'A number of years ago, I was introduced to a family consisting of mum, dad and three children. All five of them were qualified practitioners. Mum and dad had paid for their three children to qualify and their accountant had not suggested any way of mitigating the cost. The parents had borne all of the training costs out of their after tax income – something in excess of £60,000, whereas all of this could have legitimately been a business expense.'

Top tip

Bursaries

Students from low-income families, or those having financial problems, may be eligible for grants or bursaries offered by the colleges or their validating universities. These can vary from a few hundred pounds to a full year's fees so it is definitely worth asking to see if these are available.

Implications of borrowing

Apart from the obvious implication that you have to pay the money back at some point, there may or may not be tax implications. As a general rule, the costs of acquiring an initial skill to enable you to commence a trade or a profession are not allowable. However, if you are already qualified in an allied profession *and* trading in that profession, then you may be able to claim these course costs under Continuing Professional Development (CPD), see Chapter 12.

When contacting HM Revenue & Customs (HMRC) regarding CPD remember that if you can demonstrate that you already know a reasonable amount about the various aspects of the training, then it can be considered as CPD.

Repaying loans

Student loans are repaid in one of three ways (most chiropractors are self-employed so the first option rarely comes into play):

1.   By deduction from your salary (if you are employed)
2.   By direct payment with your self-assessment tax payment
3.   By voluntary direct payment

Let us say that your student loan 'enters repayment' on 6 April following qualification. What does this mean in real terms? Assume you qualify in July 2017, your loan will enter repayment from 6 April 2018 and you may have to make a payment towards this with your income tax payment, which will fall due on 31 January 2020.

You only have to make a student loan repayment if your taxable income is more than £21,000 for the year. Any repayment is calculated as 9% of your income over this figure. So if you made a profit of £30,000 you would make a student loan repayment of £810. Given that your student loan debt is likely to be in the region of £30,000, repaying £810 won't make much of a hole in it.

Top tip

Do not forget that interest will be added to a student loan and will be calculated at the rate of inflation plus 3% while you are studying, and then somewhere between the rate of inflation and the rate of inflation plus 3% once you have graduated, dependent upon your income each year. Any part of your student loan still outstanding 30 years after the date it enters repayment will automatically be wiped out.

Living costs

If you are going to be moving away from home then you need to consider the cost of renting accommodation close to where you are studying. The cost will vary depending on which college you choose. If you are studying at weekends you will most likely be based at your home and so you need to work out the cost of travelling as well as perhaps some bed-and-breakfast accommodation. Sometimes, when students get to know each other, they can share accommodation and this can keep the costs down.

As a full-time student you will be exempt from paying council tax, and you may also be able to get special deals on home insurance, mobile phones and travel, which can save you money. There are plenty of websites that list some of the best deals. (See Useful resources).

Once you have graduated

New chiropractic graduates deserve a nightly pat on the back – it is the road less travelled! Once you have actually received your graduate certificate and your General Chiropractic Council registration (that you will have applied for following graduation), plus your professional indemnity insurance policy, you will then need to contact the taxman. If you are the lucky recipient of a PAYE job offer in a clinic then you must liaise with the management of the clinic, present them with any previous employment forms and make sure that you are incorporated onto the payroll. If, like the majority of newly qualified chiropractors, you are setting up as a self-employed practitioner, you will need to register this information with HMRC.

If you plan to be self-employed, you will need to understand how to manage your finances. This will include registering with HMRC, keeping detailed records, ensuring you have receipts for any expenditure, as well as understanding tax rates, NI contributions and the deadlines to which you must submit information to HMRC. This sounds daunting, but it is achievable and HMRC offers a wealth of information to support you (see *Useful resources*).

Top tip

If you are going to assume self-employed status, you have a window of three months from the date of commencement to advise HMRC that you are self-employed. Failure to do so may make you liable to a fine of up to £100.

Professional fees

You will have a number of professional obligations once you graduate, and these are the 'cost of doing business'. Registering with the General Chiropractic Council (GCC) is a 'must' so that you can practise as a chiropractor. The current registration fee for a new graduate is £750 a year, and £800 thereafter. The GCC has given a commitment to reduce this fee over the next few years, but in the meantime this is the sum you will need to budget.

You are strongly advised to become a member of one of the chiropractic professional associations. They will be your 'trade union' and will support you in your practice life by providing appropriate insurance, record cards, promotional materials, conferences and other continuing professional development events. The cost of joining varies from association to association but all will give you discounts in your early years until you establish your practice.

The College of Chiropractors (CoC) is another organisation you should consider joining to ensure that you are part of the postgraduate activities of the profession. This will cost you less than £300 a year and, among many other advantages, will provide you with discounted CPD and a structure within which to progress your career (see Chapter 12).

Chapter summary

There is no getting away from the fact that you will have to pay to become a chiropractor and you will need to discipline yourself to manage your incoming and outgoings. Finances can seem intimidating, but the important thing is to plan so that money worries are not a distraction from enjoying yourself during your time at college.

Key points

- Contact Student Finance England or Wales and establish your entitlement to loans and grants. See what other funding routes apply.
- Consider whether there are any routes for the costs of your study to be treated as tax deductions either for you or for someone else.
- Make sure you register with HMRC post-graduation in a timely fashion.
- Think about employing a bookkeeper or accountant to help you manage your finances.

Useful resources

Business education and support team events: www.hmrc.gov.uk/bst/advice-team-events/work1.htm

Educational grants search tool: www.family-action.org.uk

HRMC: Information on being self-employed: www.hmrc.gov.uk/selfemployed/index.shtml

National Association of Student Money Advisers: www.nasma.org.uk

Paying back loans: www.direct.gov.uk/en/educationandlearning/universityandhighereducation/studentfinance/repayingstudentloanscoursesstarting from1998/dg_10034866

Student Finance England: www.studentfinance.direct.gov.uk/portal/page?_pageid=153,4680119&_dad=portal&_schema=PORTAL

Student Finance Wales: www.studentfinancewales.co.uk/portal/page?_pageid=616,6200692&_dad=portal&_schema=PORTAL

Student resources: www.students.com

Student specific sites:
www.savethestudent.org
www.studentcashpoint.co.uk
www.mystudentbills.com

Chapter 8

Chiropractic as a second career – is it too late for me to train?

Valerie S Pennacchio and
Christina Cunliffe

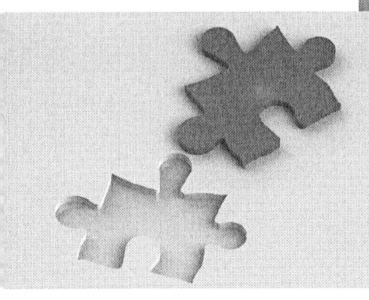

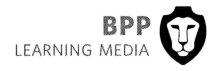

As with all high-demand careers, chiropractic can truly be seen as a lifestyle choice – a lifestyle that helps people on their pathway to health! So you have a question to answer: is chiropractic the right career for you at this time in your life? Perhaps at the moment you are sitting at a desk working in an office. Maybe you enjoy some of what you do at work but are ready for a change. Possibly you have been made redundant or are coming up for early retirement but are not yet ready to give up work altogether. All in all, the chances are that your current lifestyle no longer suits you. As a chiropractor your lifestyle will be very different. You will almost certainly be self-employed and able to choose how and when you want to practise. Essentially, you will be in control of your own destiny.

Assess your skills – time for a different lifestyle?

The decision to change your career is always a complicated one, as what you will really be doing is changing your life and it will impact not only on you but also on your family. However, if you liked jigsaw puzzles or 'connect-the-dots' games as a child, and as an adult you are a life-long learner, intrigued by how the pieces of a person's life intertwine, then the study of chiropractic could be for you.

What are you looking for in a second career?

Once you have investigated the details about a career in chiropractic, explore you, your needs and your aspirations. Start by you reflecting on a few questions. We are often harder on ourselves than we should be, so do not stop with your own reflections. Seek the opinions and thoughts of your friends, family and work colleagues. Here are few questions to get you started:

- What drives or inspires you?
- Do you like working with people?
- Do you like using your hands and making things work?
- Why are you thinking about a career change?
- Are you unhappy in your current job or career?
- What is it that you like about what you are doing and what is it you do not like?
- What do you want from your life's work (career)?
- What has attracted you to consider chiropractic as a career?
- What are your personal goals for the short, medium and long term?

'Since I was helped by a chiropractor I have always wanted to do the same for others. There was no way that I could give up my job in order to train so being able to do some of my studying through distance learning meant that I could manage my work and family commitments around my college requirements. It made it possible for my dream to come true.' **Mature student – Year 2**

Will chiropractic suit me?

The beauty of a career in chiropractic is that it can satisfy a wide range of personalities and interests, from the person who wants to work with patients all day or the person motivated to inspire others through teaching within a chiropractic educational institution, to those that want to contribute to the body of knowledge in healthcare and have research in their sights.

As a mature entrant to the profession, you will be interested in how you can manage your new career around your other commitments. As the majority of chiropractors are self-employed, you can choose to work a full five days a week or, say, only three days a week to let you play golf. You can also choose to work only mornings and evenings when your children are at school or in bed. It is really up to you.

Of course, the more you work the more you will earn, so you do need to consider how much you are taking home at the moment. 'Money makes the world go around', so be honest and look long and hard at what your financial needs might be. Chiropractic is certainly a profession that offers a very good earning potential, but of course that does not happen immediately upon graduation. You will probably want to become a chiropractor because of your desire to help people, but chiropractic is also a business. Make sure that the programme you choose provides you with the practice-building skills you need to earn your living.

Capitalising on your strengths – what are you good at?

People are more likely to enjoy their job when they are good at what they are doing and when they are passionate about why they are doing it. A career in chiropractic will involve a great deal of contact with people: patients, families, carers and other healthcare professionals. You certainly do not have to be best friends with every person you come in contact with but genuinely liking people will be a plus. The interpersonal skills you have acquired throughout your life will be second nature to you in your new career.

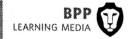

Chiropractic is a hands-on profession and much of your learning will come through your active participation. You may be worried that you are not 'touchy-feely' enough to be a chiropractor as your day job involves little or no physical contact with others. Do not be concerned, as many people who embark on a career in chiropractic start off feeling just the same way. 'Second career chiropractors' come from many different professions: accountancy, IT, marketing, teaching, the armed forces and office workers, and you will be supported to develop the necessary skills of connection and touch during your training.

'When I made my application to study to be a chiropractor, I had spent most of my working life in an office. I was a little concerned about my ability to develop the hands-on skills needed to be a good chiropractor. I needn't have worried. At my interview I was told that I had a nice firm handshake and that my typing skills meant that my fingers were mobile and used to finding the keys with accuracy. The regular practical sessions throughout the course have been brilliant in helping me develop my skills of touch. I can't wait to start working in clinic with real patients and putting my new skills to good use.'
Mature student – Year 1

Building on your existing career

You may already be in a health-related career and are looking for something more challenging. If you are a massage or beauty therapist or a fitness trainer, for example, you already have knowledge of anatomy and physiology plus skills in dealing with people that you can transfer to a chiropractic programme. Nurses also have great people skills and a deep knowledge of the human body but perhaps do not find their profession as rewarding as it once was.

Choosing to study such an intricate and amazing subject as the human body in health and disease can seem incredibly daunting, especially if you have been out of education for a while. Sometimes mature students are concerned that their brain will not re-engage with study again and that they will not reach the standards required. However, if you take things one topic at time you will come to realise that knowledge slowly builds and, as long as your studies are properly structured, you will soon realise that you are taking on board more and more complex situations as the programme progresses.

Routine or variety?

Because human beings are so diverse, there is not a lot of routine in the average working day of a chiropractor. Every patient is unique so, although many of the elements of your practice may be similar, variety will be the order of the day. When looking at a change of career this aspect can seem very attractive. Some chiropractors will also vary their practice by working with children, older people, sports people or even animals (see Chapters 14 and 15) and this is what makes chiropractic interesting, enjoyable and rewarding.

Case study

Max (son of Quentin Willson) was born in April 1998 after a very difficult labour. The umbilical cord was wrapped twice around Max's neck and he had to be delivered quickly. Quentin and Michaela (the mother) soon noticed that Max was not developing in the same way that his elder sister, Mercedes, had done seven years previously. His eyes did not focus and his hand movements were more unco-ordinated compared with his contemporaries. Max was unable to concentrate, he was hyperactive, demanding and every childhood hurdle was twice as difficult as it had been for his sister. He wore nappies until he was four, was impossible to wean from the bottle and had never slept through the night.

When Max went to school, the couple began to seek help. They consulted both state and private health professionals, trying to discover what was wrong with their son and were given diagnoses, including dyspraxia and dyslexia. They even began to think that Max was autistic. Quentin and Michaela were at the point of putting Max on Ritalin, the drug used to treat children with attention deficit hyperactivity disorders, when they met a mother who had been observing Max at a birthday party and who suggested that he should see a chiropractor, Deirdre Edwards.

Though deeply sceptical, the Willsons felt that they had nothing to lose in crossing yet another treatment off their list. Deirdre remembers Michaela coming into her practice with an air of resignation and exhaustion, while Max wreaked havoc in the waiting room. Deirdre put him through a range of assessments and discovered that he was delayed in several areas. But she did manage to make eye contact, which suggested to her that he did not have severe autism. Once she had checked that it was safe to give chiropractic help, Deirdre began to treat Max. She found that four of his seven neck bones were severely misaligned and that this was affecting the natural nerve function throughout his body.

 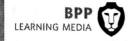

The Willsons remember the treatment not hurting Max at all, and that night he slept continuously until the morning for the first time since his birth. Deirdre continued to see Max about once a week for the first month, and then every ten to 14 days. His speech, eating and abilities quickly improved to the point where he now only visits her once a month. Max now 'sleeps like a log' and has lost all his 'weirdness', according to his father. He no longer has a classroom assistant and has moved to a village state school where he is flourishing.

> 'This is an unimpeachable case history from a man who did not believe in chiropractic. We have to raise awareness, because it worked so thoroughly for my son and changed his life and ours. If I can help just one child that is going through what we went through, then that is my reward.' (Quentin Willson)

Do you have the qualities to be a good chiropractor?

Some of the most important qualities that make a good chiropractor are a sincere desire to help people, being a good communicator and working well in a team environment. Expect to team up with, not only your patients, but other healthcare professionals including chiropractors, physiotherapists, GPs, consultants and occupational health therapists. Are you capable of making decisions under pressure? Can you think quickly and creatively?

Top tip

It will be important to be able to draw on all that you have learned to offer solutions to a patient's healthcare needs. If you have had another career before chiropractic, the life skills that you have acquired will stand you in very good stead.

You have what it takes to be a chiropractor – what next?

Do not be concerned that the chiropractic colleges will not accept you as a mature applicant. When they are considering applications, they will always take into account your life experiences and give you credit for prior experience and learning (known as APEL). All of the colleges also run pathway or access programmes to help you acquire the necessary basic requirements to enrol (see Chapter 6). Some colleges, like the McTimoney College of Chiropractic, have a programme that is particularly geared towards encouraging mature learners and those changing career. Their five-year master's programme is run predominantly at weekends and through spring and summer schools to allow you to manage your training alongside your existing work and family commitments.

> 'I have been interested in becoming a chiropractor for a while. But as I co-own a business and home-school a teenager I didn't see how I could do it. To say my life is busy is an understatement. But I still had this goal. When I found there was a course that catered for people like me, I thought that this might be the way. Having started the programme I can highly recommend it. I've also thoroughly enjoyed the comradeship of the many mature students on my course.'
> **Mature student – Year 1**

Having the appropriate grades and academic credentials to apply to chiropractic college is an obvious requirement, however, do not underestimate the importance of the non-academic aspects of your application. Extra-curricular activities support a person pursuing any career, and as a mature applicant you will probably be well ahead of the game in this respect

Chiropractic colleges are looking for well-rounded, sociable people who contribute positively to their learning environment as well as to the community in general. Participating in extra-curricular activities is a great way to demonstrate these qualities. It is also an excellent way to develop a practical approach to a work-life balance. That balance will be a integral part of your success in both your chiropractic studies and beyond.

Chapter summary

When you are already established in your career, thinking about a change of direction is a huge decision and not one to be taken lightly. But if you are thinking about a new focus in life, it is probably because you are dissatisfied with what you are doing now. Becoming a chiropractor will mean that you can regain a purpose in life and there is nothing more rewarding than knowing that you were instrumental in helping another person on the road to recovery and health. Many people every year decide to change careers and it is never too late to retrain.

Key points

- Consider the things you like and do not like about your current job and see if chiropractic can provide what is lacking.

- Do not be put off by your lack of academic qualifications as life experience is taken into account.

- Teamwork, leadership and communication skills are qualities that you will be able to evidence through your previous career.

- Consider a training programme that is focused towards mature learners.

- Chiropractic will provide you with a stimulating and rewarding new career.

Useful resources

Engaging adult learners: www.aare.edu.au/06pap/kni06315.pdf

The British Education System: www.blueu.co.uk/maturestudent.php

The Higher Education Academy:
www.heacademy.ac.uk/assets/EvidenceNet/Syntheses/wp_mature_learners_synthesis_on_template_updated_090310.pdf

Universities & Colleges Admissions Service:
www.ucas.com/students/wheretostart/maturestudents

Chapter 9

What is life like as a student chiropractor?

Mary Young

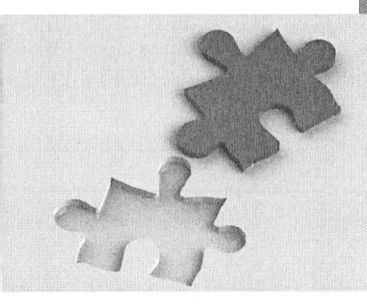

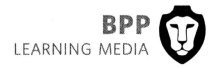

A master's in Chiropractic is not a degree you are likely to study just in order to enjoy the 'university experience'. It is a vocational course, leading not just to a qualification, but to a profession that lasts a lifetime. The decision to embark on this particular path is one you will consider very carefully.

Pre-qualifications

When you imagine being a manual therapist, it is easy to focus on the hands-on treatment in a clinic room that you might have seen or experienced. Yet there is no getting away from the fact that qualifying as a chiropractor involves a great deal of 'hard' science. It is by understanding the way the body works that chiropractors are able to make the right intervention with their hands. The manual techniques are taught during the courses, but it is necessary for students to have a basic background in science before they start. Biology and chemistry are the most relevant A level subjects, but do not despair if you have not chosen to study these subjects. There are one-year access courses available to get you to where you need to be (see Chapters 5 and 6).

Books and equipment

From day one, everything you are taught on a chiropractic programme builds towards what you need to know as a practising chiropractor. The days of learning something for an exam and then forgetting it forever are over! It may not be surprising to know that there are some books you will use all the way through the programme and, if you can, it is probably best to buy them early on, maximising page-turns per pound. One shock to the system can be that academic books are in a different price range from the paperbacks we take on holiday, and over time you will get used to the fact that you might not get change from £50 when you add to your library. For a book that you will refer to regularly for the next twenty years or so this is not so bad, but choose carefully before you invest.

College libraries are a godsend while you are saving, and for reference books that you will use only once or twice. Being registered as a student also gives you access to the world of online journals (see Useful resources), which is where the cutting edge of published research is available to you. As your studies progress, being able to access journal articles in a particular field becomes more important in addition to the core information that the textbooks give you. You will also be able to gain access to a Virtual Learning Environment (VLE) where study materials and college communications are posted, whether you are on campus or studying at home.

College lectures

Most of the contact time spent at college takes the form of lectures. They are the traditional way to deliver a large amount of material to a large group of people. Different lecturers have different styles and some sessions are more interactive than others, but essentially there will be many hours of sitting in a lecture room trying to keep up with whoever is talking to you about their subject (see Chapter 9).

Top tips

It can difficult to keep your brain in 'receive' mode for long periods during lectures, and there are various ways to maximise the amount you retain:

- Taking notes is really helpful: not only does it keep you awake, it also allows you to add clarifying comments and personalise any handouts that are provided.

- You can flag any topics that you realise you need to make sure of afterwards.

- Your lecture 'scribbles' will act as prompts when you come to review the lecture material, and because there is not enough time for your lecturer to repeat things (something you might be used to from your experience in school), you *will* have to review what has been said in order to get it into your long-term memory.

Studying systematically

People learn new information permanently by means of the following process: first they hear or read it, then they understand it and then they repeat it a number of times. Lectures only cover the first and, possibly, the second of these steps. One of the features of post-A level education is that reviewing and reflecting on the material provided in lectures is a significant and crucial part of the process. If you are disciplined and allocate time to this review and reflection every week, you will be in the best position to make sense of the contents of the next lecture, which will start from where the last one left off.

Self-directed study is a really important part of the learning process and not simply a necessary evil to help you pass exams. You will be gaining an education, not just attending a training course, and as you develop as a chiropractor you have the chance to develop your own

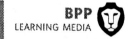

personal philosophy. You need to fit any new material into a matrix of understanding if you want to remember and use it, and the particular network of information that you create is very personal, reflecting your own interests and experience. Taking an active role in what you learn, such as looking up a topic in a book or on the internet in order to find the key that makes it relevant for you, allows you to shape your learning and thus your own mind. It also lets you spot and query any dubious information that you come across during your research, which is a handy skill to have ready when trawling the internet!

Practical sessions

As well as the necessary theoretical study, you will have practical sessions throughout your programme, in which the hands-on element of the chiropractor's work is taught. For many students this is a new experience, but it does not take long for confidence to develop as the various techniques become familiar and physical contact with your fellow students becomes normal. Tutors will demonstrate each technique for you, talking through the desired positioning both of the patient and of the chiropractor, the mechanics of the adjustment and the reasoning behind all the specific instructions (see Chapter 11).

You will then try out what you have been shown, usually in pairs, with tutors at the ready to offer guidance. Practical sessions are where you begin to develop the motor skills that are the tools of the chiropractor's trade. They ingrain in you safe patient handling and they introduce you to your future as a chiropractor. At first, the tunics you wear for practical sessions may feel awkward, but very soon they become a symbol of your new professional role. Practical sessions will be some of the most demanding days of your course because they require you to expose yourself constantly to constructive criticism, but they are also some of the most rewarding. Attempting an adjustment for the tenth time and having it suddenly work for the first time is an amazingly satisfying moment.

'It has been an amazing experience, and surrounding the utter excitement of what the future holds, is a degree of sadness with having to say goodbye to all those who have enriched this journey. Thank you also to my family and friends for their patience, understanding and continuing support.' **New chiropractor at graduation**

Practising techniques

As well as lectures, you need to study: on top of practical sessions, you need to practise. You cannot be a good chiropractor if you do not practise your techniques; repeating the positions and movements is the only way you can train your muscles to be there for you when you need to exert a certain force in the correct direction at the right speed. Eventually, the set-up becomes second nature and your conscious brain is freed to interpret the feedback your hands are receiving from the patient. As a student, you cannot practise on unsuspecting bodies unsupervised, but you can do a great deal on your own. Think of the drill martial artists repeat, without contact, but always improving the speed, accuracy and reliability of their manoeuvres. This is what you will need to do so that you are in control of your muscles.

Top tip

Nothing but practise can get you to the stage where you are no longer just 'going through the motions', but you have reached a stage where you can feel enough and engage with the patient's body sufficiently to make an effective adjustment in a safe way.

Assessment methods

We all work better to deadlines, and the programme is therefore punctuated by dates on which you need to demonstrate your understanding of the essentials. A variety of assessment methods are used, which means that even those who find one or other method more challenging have a chance to perform in other ways too. Unseen exams are the main method of assessment, and they do become less terrifying as time goes on! The better prepared you are, the more you will enjoy them. Some modules require submission of an essay instead, particularly where the content of the course requires discussion or interpretation. Preparing these assignments develops writing skills and teaches you to research and reference your work in a professional way. These are essential skills to develop before submitting the major piece of coursework: the research dissertation (see Chapter 16).

In practical exams, your every move is assessed for safety and effectiveness as you demonstrate how you would treat a patient. These exams do become less frightening in time, and they test whether or not your practice has secured the chiropractic techniques in your subconscious so that you can perform them under stress. As always, preparation leads to success.

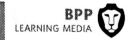

Clinic preparation

The early years of study are pre-clinical and classroom-based. Throughout, however, the vocational nature of the programme is kept in mind, as you will not only relate your theoretical learning to clinical situations but you will also be encouraged to spend time observing chiropractors (both qualified and final-year students) as they work. This is a valuable chance to acclimatise to the clinic environment long before the pressure to perform with a patient is added, and it means that the transition to working in clinic is that little bit more straightforward. You will see many and varied styles during observation and the process of reflection is another way in which you build your own approach as time goes on.

'Strength, hard work and determination are a few of the many words to describe what was required to achieve this degree, all of which has been made possible by the guidance and support provided by everybody at the college.' **New graduate**

Supervised clinic

Before you graduate, the final stage of your degree programme is an extended period working in a supervised clinic. This is the point at which your ambition of practising as a chiropractor begins to take shape. You assess and treat your own patients in a safe environment under the supervision of an experienced chiropractor. Rather than being sent out into the world with theoretical knowledge but with no experience of how to use it (like the classic university graduate!), you have the chance to continue to learn as you apply your knowledge and hone your technical, diagnostic and patient communication skills. By the time you graduate as a chiropractor, you will be ready to add value to the community by working effectively on your patients.

Peer support

Chiropractor training is not an easy option. The programme is long and requires you to be good with your brain and also with your hands. Throughout the training, you have to be ready to challenge your own ideas about the world and about yourself, and you have to be prepared to work harder than ever before to develop your skills. Throughout these years of hard study, however, support is available. All your fellow students are travelling the same rocky road and so they will understand what you face. A real community develops, in which people quickly learn not only to give help to any fellow student but also, importantly, to ask for it without embarrassment. Whether the student culture of teamwork and support is generated by the degree programme, or whether people who choose chiropractic training are naturally good people, the college environment certainly allows these virtues to flourish in a remarkable way.

Case study: New chiropractic graduate

'My time at chiropractic college brought me the bonus of new friends that supported me through the tough times, and who studied, drank, camped, partied, and laughed together. One of the things I loved most about the course was the contact it gave me with people from so many different walks of life: we had school leavers, ex-military personnel, para-medics, "new age" spiritual types who wanted an official stamp on their healing abilities, divorced mothers wanting a second chance – and everyone in between. The camaraderie that you get on a chiropractic course cannot be understated – you experience such highs and lows together, and you even lose your embarrassment about taking your clothes off in front of each other in practical sessions – always an ice-breaker! I am grateful to every one of them for helping me make it such a memorable and priceless journey.'

Chapter summary

Every qualified chiropractor has been a student at some stage of course; trying to fix facts in their memory or finding the right angle for an effective adjustment. Your tutors and supervisors can remember being in your position and they are ready to offer encouragement when you need it. The moment you embark on a chiropractic programme you become part of the chiropractic community and you will find that any chiropractor, anywhere, is pleased to help. One day you will do the same for the next generation of students.

Key points

- Being a chiropractor is a way of life, not just a job.
- You will be expected to be professional, even when off-duty.
- You will discover as much about yourself as you will about the subjects being taught.
- The courses are demanding and, for that reason, highly rewarding.
- If you can work hard and want to achieve something great, then your decision to enroll could be the best one you have ever made.

Useful resources

BioMedNet: www.biomedcentral.com

National Union of Students: www.nus.org.uk

PubMed: www.ncbi.nlm.nih.gov/pubmed

Science Direct: www.sciencedirect.com

Student sites: www.studentbeans.com, www.thestudentroom.co.uk

Chapter 10

Chiropractic study
– what will I learn?

Gill Amos

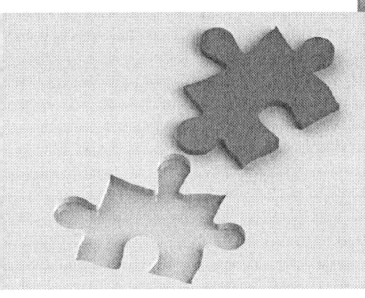

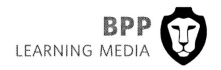

As with any new subject that you learn, you have to start with the basics. Individual colleges will do things in different ways, of course, and perhaps amalgamate modules or call them different names, but all colleges have to fulfil the criteria of the General Chiropractic Council (GCC) in order for their programmes to be accepted and recognised. Whatever chiropractic college you decide to attend, you will get all the necessary knowledge, understanding and skills for your chosen career.

It will come as no surprise to you that your early years will be spent acquiring knowledge and understanding of the basic sciences, such as anatomy, physiology and biochemistry. Next you will build on this and see how the knowledge can be applied and then put into a clinical context, for example, subjects such as behavioural science, clinical neurology and differential diagnosis. You will learn about the history of chiropractic and how it fits within the wider modern healthcare system – as well as acquainting yourself with your legal and ethical responsibilities as a chiropractor. Finally, you will undertake clinical training (see Chapter 11).

Degree programme outcomes

During the degree course students must meet set standards (known as programme outcomes) for the following areas of knowledge and skill:

- Those that form the basis of chiropractic, including history, theory and principles of chiropractic
- Normal and abnormal structure and functioning of the human body and the range of presenting conditions
- Research and evaluation
- Case / patient assessment
- Chiropractic care
- Communication with patients and other healthcare professionals
- Independent primary healthcare practice
- Professional accountability and the protection of patients according to GCC standards

---

Practical modules

As chiropractic involves placing your hands on patients and making adjustments, you will be taught how to assess the body and apply the relevant adjustments. These practical modules will be studied throughout the programme to ensure that your skills develop over time (see Chapter 11). Another topic that is taught from the outset of each programme is research (see Chapter 16). It is through research that you will be able to learn how to critically evaluate scientific evidence, which will ultimately improve your practice.

Basic sciences

You will find that you need to acquire a lot of knowledge to understand how the body works. Sometimes called 'human structure and function', the basic sciences are the underpinning modules upon which everything else builds.

Anatomy

The study of anatomy will introduce you to the organisational levels of the human body as well as the anatomical language used. This will give you an understanding of where the muscles, bones, nerves and blood vessels are found in relation to each other as well as a detailed understanding of the systems of the body, for example, the nervous system and the cardiovascular system. Histology, which is the anatomical study of the microscopic structure of the body, will also be covered. It is important that you can recognise what is normal and abnormal anatomy in the body. Particular attention will be paid to surface anatomy, which helps with palpation.

> 'If I were to give one bit of advice to first year students, it would be to study their anatomy, then some anatomy and then some more anatomy. Without a full knowledge of the structure of the human body you will not understand the physiology and function to be able to eventually diagnose and evaluate musculoskeletal conditions in the future. Use the excellent lectures, facilities and practical time to learn, collate and ask questions!' **Final-year chiropractic student**

Physiology

Physiology is the study of the body's regulatory processes, such as temperature and pH regulation, breathing, metabolism or any other process that keeps the body alive. Each of the systems of the body will be covered, with an emphasis on homeostasis (the means by which the body maintains internal equilibrium). Particular attention will be paid to the physiology of the muscular and skeletal systems.

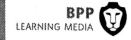

Biochemistry

Biochemistry is the study of how chemicals behave within the body. As well as the underlying function of the components of cells, this module will give you an understanding of the way the body uses and metabolises biomolecules such as sugars, fats, proteins and amino acids. This will enable you to advise patients on more efficient ways of exercising, for example.

Biomechanics

Biomechanics goes hand-in-hand with anatomy and is very important for the adjusting skills that you will learn later in the programme. It is the study of the mechanics of a living body, especially of the forces exerted by muscles and the effect of gravity on the skeleton. You will gain an understanding of the basic engineering principles and concepts in physics that apply to the human musculoskeletal system, particularly the concept that 'structure equals function'. Each of the major joints of the body will be covered with an emphasis on assessment of function.

'It was only later in the programme that I realised how important biomechanics was. I would come across a case and think, "Oh yes, we covered that in biomechanics". Its principles crop up throughout the programme.' **Chiropractic student**

Applied and clinical sciences

During the intermediate years, the applied and clinical science subjects you will learn about will include pathology, pharmacology, behavioural science, imaging, musculoskeletal medicine, clinical neurology, general medicine and differential diagnosis. Sometimes these are exactly what the modules will be called, or the subject matter might be combined under more general clinic science topics. These are the key areas, however, that will underpin your clinical thinking.

Pathology

Pathology is the study of disease and disease processes. This is what happens when the body starts to dysfunction and how you recognise it. To begin with you will be taught the mechanisms of disease and the signs and symptoms associated with pathological processes. You will also cover pathology of the systems of the body, for example, the cardiovascular and respiratory systems. This will be taught using case studies to illustrate the underlying pathology of common clinical conditions that you are likely to encounter as a chiropractor.

Pharmacology

Pharmacology is the study of drugs and their effects on the body. Chiropractors do not prescribe drugs, but nevertheless you need to know about them as many of your patients will be on one or more medications that might affect your chiropractic care. You will learn about the classification of drugs in everyday use, including the common prescription and non-prescription therapeutic drugs. An important aspect of this subject is the indications for use of drugs and the possible side-effects. You will also gain an understanding of how other remedies (such as homeopathic and herbal) could be used to address various disorders.

Top tip

Throughout training in pharmacology, you will be given an awareness of the relevance and implications of common drugs that chiropractors need to be aware of. For example, patients who are taking anticoagulant drugs should be treated with caution, and some commonly prescribed drugs to reduce cholesterol can cause muscular aches and pains as a side effect.

Behavioural science

In the context of a chiropractic programme, behavioural science is concerned with the basic concepts of psychology and how this may impact on clinical chiropractic practice. It is one of the tools to help you manage your patients in your clinic. For example, the psychology of sport is important as you will have patients in your practice who may not listen to your advice to stop jogging or playing tennis or golf for a few weeks until their problem resolves. You will gain an understanding of the theories underpinning health psychology and about how relevant psychological models might inform your own practice. Patients who are in pain, for example, evolve different coping strategies that might impact not only on their family and work, but also on your chiropractic care. You will also gain the means to recognise the major psychological disorders and how to implement referral protocols when necessary.

Imaging

Where chiropractic is concerned, medical images are primarily used to help identify any underlying pathological conditions and to determine whether there is any reason why you should not adjust a patient. This subject is often integrated across the programme as images can help

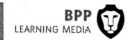

you visualise anatomy at the beginning of your studies as well as enable you to recognise pathological processes later on.

You will gain an understanding of the physical principles involved in the formation of medical images, as well as the statutory requirements relating to the role of the referrer and practitioner involved in all imaging procedures. The purpose of the different types of imaging used commonly in chiropractic practice and the associated risks or benefits of such imaging will also be outlined. With the use of problem-based learning and case-centred scenarios, this will allow you to appreciate the use of radiographic and special imaging in the context of patient management, referral and assessment.

Musculoskeletal medicine

It is well understood that chiropractic has an effect on the musculoskeletal system, and this is another area where the body can dysfunction. You will be introduced to the clinical features of common disorders of the musculoskeletal system and the main treatments used by the medical profession to manage these disorders. On a practical level, it will teach you how to clinically assess the musculoskeletal system and how to interpret the available information to allow you to diagnose common disorders of this system. This, in turn, will help you to set realistic goals for patients with regard to how quickly they are likely to respond to treatment given different presenting conditions.

Neuroscience and clinical neurology

Chiropractic affects the nervous system as well as the musculoskeletal system and that is why it is often referred to as a neuro-musculoskeletal intervention. It is essential, therefore, that you have a good understanding of this important system. Neuroscience will give you an introduction to the structure and function of the nervous system and impart an understanding of the scientific basis and significance of neurological testing and the pathophysiology of common neurological conditions.

You might have heard the term 'sciatica', for example, or know of someone who has suffered from shooting pains, tingling or numbness in the legs. Clinical neurology will equip you with the practical skills and theoretical knowledge to diagnose common neurological disorders like this that you are likely to encounter as a chiropractor and enable you to manage them appropriately. It will also allow you to recognise more serious neurological conditions that fall outside the purview of chiropractic and how to refer to neurological specialists in such cases.

General medicine

A chiropractor's first concern is to find out what is wrong. They will also check for signs of any serious conditions for which a patient would need to go to their GP or to a hospital.

As with musculoskeletal medicine and clinical neurology, general medicine will give you the knowledge and skills to understand common presentations of disorders and pathologies that you might encounter in the patients that present in a chiropractic clinic: conditions affecting the gastrointestinal, cardiovascular or endocrine systems, for example. You will gain an understanding of the general principles of nutrition and how diet and deficiency influence the onset of disease (a deficiency in Vitamin D, for example, leads to rickets in children). This helps you to recognise when patients may not be receiving suitable nutrition.

Some conditions present in specific populations (children, the elderly or pregnant women, for example) and so the common disease processes that apply to particular patient groups will be covered. Case studies are often used to illustrate the underlying pathology of common clinical conditions and systemic diseases, such as diabetes, that you are likely to encounter as a chiropractor.

> 'Musculoskeletal medicine and differential diagnosis – what amazing subjects and so relevant to what we do as chiropractors – all linked together with general medicine and underpinning my diagnostic approach to patients on a day-to-day basis in clinic.' **Chiropractic student**

Differential diagnosis

Before chiropractors adjust patients, they must first determine whether it is safe to do so. This is done by a process of considering the possible causes for the patient's condition and ruling out any serious pathological processes or 'red flags', as they are known. This process is called differential diagnosis. You will be taught the processes involved in identifying the key diagnostic features of a case presentation as well as how to assess whether a patient is safe to treat. Referral processes, if needed, will also be covered to help you refine your differential diagnosis and to manage the patient accordingly. Differential diagnosis relies heavily on problem-based learning and case-centred scenarios.

BPP
LEARNING MEDIA

Case study

A patient presents with pain and tingling down the inside of their left arm. The pain and tingling could be because they are experiencing a heart attack, or because they have an irritated nerve in their neck that serves this part of the arm. By taking a clear history (during which you consider the age and lifestyle of the patient, the mode of onset, the frequency and the nature of the symptoms) and by carrying out a physical examination, you will be well equipped to determine whether the patient has a serious cardiovascular condition (a red flag for referral) or a neuro-musculoskeletal condition (perhaps a 'trapped nerve') that you can treat with chiropractic.

> *'Chiropractors take an integrated and holistic approach to the health needs of their patients, considering physical, psychological and social factors. They provide care and support by reducing pain and disability and by restoring normal function to people with neuro-musculoskeletal disorders.'* (General Chiropractic Council, 2012)

Contemporary healthcare

All of the colleges will give you a grounding in the history of medicine and chiropractic and how it fits within healthcare models worldwide and their differing philosophies and approaches. The chiropractic profession is very diverse, with a wide variety of techniques on offer and different ways or models of practising. For example, patients may come to see you only when they have symptoms, or they may choose to come on a regular basis to aid their ongoing wellbeing and to help prevent future problems. This is similar to a patient's attendance at their dentist or optometrist: they either wait until they have a toothache or cannot see clearly, or they attend for regular checkups. Some colleges will include philosophy modules that will help you explore and consider your own views around healthcare and also how you yourself want to practise as a chiropractor.

Definition

'**Health** is a state of complete physical, mental and social wellbeing and not merely the absence of disease or infirmity.' (World Health Organisation, 1948)

As a chiropractor in the UK, you will be required to abide by the *Code of Practice* and *Standard of Proficiency* as defined by the General Chiropractic Council (see Chapter 2). As such, you will need to understand the ethical, legal and financial implications of setting up in practice in the UK. You will need to know your responsibilities in this regard, including gaining patient consent, keeping patient information confidential and how to maintain professional boundaries.

Chapter summary

There is a lot to learn, but an important thing to remember while you are studying is that as a chiropractor you will have responsibility for the safety and care of your patients once you have graduated. Whatever the specific structure of the programme you choose, it will build year-on-year so that you start to not only understand, but also to integrate your knowledge, so that you are well placed to make clinical decisions as you start working with patients.

Key points

- Your first two years at chiropractic college will be spent mainly learning the basic sciences.

- There will be a mixture of teaching styles, varying between lectures and problem-based learning.

- Before entering the clinical stage of training, you will understand body systems and how to ensure that it is safe and appropriate to treat patients.

- You will learn how chiropractic fits into the wider healthcare model and what your ethical and legal responsibilities are.

Useful resources

Anglo-European College of Chiropractic: www.aecc.ac.uk

McTimoney College of Chiropractic: www.mctimoney-college.ac.uk

University of Glamorgan, Faculty of Health, Sport and Science: http://hesas.glam.ac.uk

References

General Chiropractic Council (2012) *What is Chiropractic?* [Online] Available at: www.gcc-uk.org/page.cfm?page_id=4&4fc=1&hi=holistic#hi [Accessed 29 July 2012]

Preamble to the Constitution of the World Health Organisation as adopted by the International Health Conference, New York, 19-22 June, 1946; signed on 22 July 1946 by the representatives of 61 states (Official Records of the World Health Organisation, no. 2, p. 100) and entered into force on 7 April 1948.

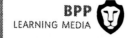

Chapter 11

Chiropractic study – practical and clinical training

Gill Amos and Christina Cunliffe

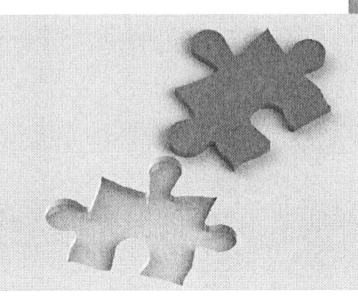

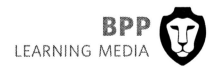

The scientific underpinning knowledge you acquire on a chiropractic programme will help you explain and understand the theories behind what you are doing in practice. Your practical studies, however, will develop the tools of your trade; the essential technique skills you will need when you are adjusting patients. When you are judged ready, you will start your clinical training working on real patients in the supervised chiropractic training clinic.

Practical studies

This is a subject that you will take in every year of your chiropractic programme before you enter your final year or years in clinic. The manual skills required for patient management and technique application take time to develop and so, early in the programme, you will be taught exercises that help you develop the skills necessary for you to deliver effective chiropractic adjustments. These exercises train the muscles in your own body so that they will respond quickly and automatically for a safe and effective adjustment.

Another important aspect is developing your skills of 'palpation'. Palpation involves 'feeling' a patient with your hands during a physical examination. This sense of connection and touch is an integral part of how chiropractors assess patients. Before you can apply an adjustment, you must first be able to detect where an input is required. This is done with careful palpation of the body, assessing for function and tone. Is the body correctly positioned and is it moving correctly? Are the muscles evenly balanced or is one side tight or warm? These are all indications that the body is not functioning correctly at a structural level.

As the practical programme progresses, you will learn to position the patient correctly and then apply your chosen adjustment with speed and precision. As with any practical skill, such as playing tennis, practice makes perfect. Throughout the programme you will be encouraged to hone your practical skills, initially on your fellow students. When you have been assessed as competent you will be able to apply them on real patients in the student clinic.

Different chiropractic techniques

There are hundreds of different specific chiropractic techniques used around the world, but all aim to remove any impediment to the body's own self-healing ability and to optimise function. Many techniques rely on what is known as a High Velocity Low Amplitude (HVLA) force application, which involves a very fast, shallow thrust into the body.

Other students are taught very light impulse techniques, while others might use cushions or blocks with wedges to make the necessary changes in the body. Some techniques incorporate the use of instruments, which may be hand-held or mounted. At chiropractic college you will be taught at least one, or a number of, technique systems that will allow you to safely and competently adjust the patients in your care. You will also be shown how to use mobilisations and soft tissue techniques as an adjunct to chiropractic adjusting.

Widely-taught techniques

One of the main technique systems taught is often referred to as 'diversified' technique. This is an HVLA approach and patients often hear a 'pop' or a 'click' as the thrust is made into the spine. Another well-known chiropractic technique is the McTimoney 'toggle torque recoil' technique used by over a quarter of the chiropractors in the UK. Based on the toggle-recoil technique used by BJ Palmer, the son of the developer of chiropractic, this is also an HVLA thrust, but employs recoil to make it even faster and lighter. As a matter of routine, this approach also addresses the pelvis, cranium and extremities as well as the spine.

Segmental approach

You will learn about different ways of approaching a specific problem. Take something simple like a patient who comes to see you with pain in the neck. You will have gone through all of your diagnostic testing and decided it is a case that will benefit from chiropractic. Probably you will find that the upper cervical vertebrae (the top two bones in the neck) are rotated to one side, and that the shoulder on that side is raised because the muscles between the neck and shoulder have become tight. If you adjust the vertebrae to reposition them, and so release the tension in the muscles, then the problem may resolve. This is known as a segmental approach – in other words you are adjusting the area where the symptom has manifested.

Postural or whole-body approach

Some chiropractors will look at the whole body because, for example, if the pelvis is tilted then this will give rise to compensations in the spine that could be the root cause of the tension in the shoulder. This, in turn, could give rise to the neck pain. This is known as a postural or whole-body approach where the chiropractor will adjust other areas, particularly the pelvis or extremities, which might ultimately be the root cause of the problem.

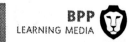

Top tip

The three chiropractic colleges teach different techniques and also differ in that they may approach chiropractic from either a more holistic or more biomechanical perspective depending on their ideology. Make sure that you ask questions when you attend an open day to be clear whether or not the approach on offer is one that resonates with your own chiropractic experiences or philosophy.

'It goes without saying that technique classes were the best bit. You learn the hands-on skills that you are going to use as a chiropractor and practise these so that they become second nature. All the technique instructors were excellent.' **Chiropractic student**

Clinical training

Your final clinic year is the culmination of all your previous learning; this is when you will integrate the knowledge and skills you have accumulated in the earlier years of study into a real clinical environment. Here you will gain experience of managing your own patient caseload under supervised conditions acting as a student practitioner / clinic intern. It is a time of great excitement as you realise you will be working at last on real patients, but at this point that you may also realise that you really should have been applying yourself to your studies an awful lot sooner!

But even though this is the moment of truth, so to speak, you will have prepared for this gradually by gaining an understanding of the clinical setting during observations in the earlier years of the programme. There is also no need to worry as you will not be allowed into clinic until you have been assessed as competent to do so.

Observation and self-reflection

In each year of the programme you will be required to undertake a certain number of hours observing in a clinical setting. This will vary depending on which programme you choose, but normally you will be observing in the student chiropractic clinic, chiropractors working in the field, and other allied healthcare professionals, such as physiotherapists. These structured observations develop through the programme as you gain greater knowledge and understanding of clinical practice. They will enable you to view chiropractic in practice and will encompass ethics, patient management and the patient-practitioner interaction.

Top tip

If you have just been learning about pharmacology in the academic part of the programme, for example, you may want to look up the various medications of the patients that come to clinic. Doing this will help reinforce how what you are learning is relevant to your practice, and it will also make it more real to you. By observing other healthcare professionals, you will gain an appreciation of the roles of other healthcare providers and their models of patient management, and also how you may interact with them once you graduate.

When you have graduated as a chiropractor, you will have to use your clinical judgment to decide on the best way in which to manage and help patients. To do this, you must be a *thinking* practitioner who is willing to develop and change practices according to your patients' needs and your own skill levels. You must also be able to embrace developments in best practice in the profession (see Chapter 16). Above all, chiropractors must be self-reflective.

A thinking profession

You will start to develop the skills of self-reflection early on in your chiropractic programme and this self-reflection underpins the observational aspect of your clinical training in particular. You will be expected to reflect on what you have seen and explore what it might mean and any consequences arising from it. This will help you to develop new perspectives in a non-judgmental way as you progress and develop as an individual, as well as a student practitioner. Self-reflection will be used to help you consider how you can satisfy your own learning needs in the student clinical setting, and of course these are essential skills for your future practice life.

Case study: Fitting the final jigsaw pieces together – new chiropractic graduate

'The final clinic year at chiropractic college was the most challenging and valuable year for me, when I could gather my knowledge from previous lectures and learning, and finally put them into practice in a professional clinic environment with patients who had real issues and conditions. Having a range of experienced, knowledgeable clinic supervisors was key to our development and ability to assess and treat our patients appropriately by questioning our thought processes and differential diagnoses. I would have happily carried on in clinic for another six months to develop my skills further, alas all good things come to an end!'

Student clinic

Many students consider this as the time when they really start to learn. As a senior student, you will have a real patient in front of you and it will be your responsibility to manage that patient's chiropractic care under supervision. All those years of study and practice will be finally put to use, as you manage your own patient caseload both safely and ethically. You will gain expertise in primary patient care, focusing on the chiropractic management of your patients, which includes assessment, diagnosis, treatment and rehabilitation. At the same time, you will develop clinical management skills, such as completing paperwork, interacting with reception staff and communicating with fellow healthcare professionals. All of this will be conducted with a patient-centred focus and in compliance with the General Chiropractic Council's *Code of Practice* and *Standard of Proficiency* (see Chapter 2).

Peer support

You will not be alone. You will be learning with a small group of other students under the careful watching eye of your clinic supervisor who is there to support and guide you. Ultimately the clinic supervisor is responsible for the safety and care of the patients that you will see, but they will want to encourage you to take more and more responsibility as your confidence and ability develops over the year you will spend in the student clinic.

Case presentations

Case presentations are an integral part of the clinical year. After you have seen a new patient for the first time and gathered their case history and examined them, you will, through a process of differential diagnosis, determine a plan of care. You will present this plan to your supervisor and other students on your clinic shift. This often leads to discussion and provides a learning opportunity for all students working with you.

In your clinical year, you will be required typically to manage a caseload of 40 new patients. It is important that you see patients from a wide spectrum of ages and presentations so that you get experience of the types of people that you are likely to see in your own practice. You will be expected to see young people, adults and the elderly. Some chiropractic colleges have a paediatric clinic where you can gain experience in working with children, though some student clinics have restrictions on students working on babies.

Patients can have conditions varying from straightforward mechanical low back pain to the complexities of scoliosis (curvature of the spine) or osteoporosis (reduced bone density). Patients often have other underlying medical conditions, such as diabetes, cataracts, a replacement hip or hypertension. Many will attend following trauma, such as a car accident or a running injury. A great many will present because they understand that chiropractic care will benefit to their ongoing health.

'I had the best time in clinic. That is not to say it was easy, far from it – the workload was full on: dissertation, case reports and publishable reports, all between clinic hours and treating patients – it was quite a challenge. But the clinic year brought it all together and made it clear why we study what we study and learn what we learn!'
Final-year student

Case study: Clinical training case – neck pain with associated headaches

John is a 41-year-old marketing manager, who attends with low-grade neck pain and associated headaches. The neck pain has come on gradually over the last month and is intermittent during the day and located at the base of the skull. The headaches started about the same time as the neck pain and feel like a band across his forehead. Initially, he had about two or three headaches a week but he now gets them daily, usually in the afternoon. John started a new job six weeks ago and is working longer hours. He is tall and his desk area has not been set up specifically for him. There are no associated symptoms in his arms. Painkillers alleviate the headache and neck pain and there is nothing remarkable in his medical history.

Supervised diagnosis:

John has 'cervicogenic' headaches due to tension in his neck, which have been brought on by poor posture while working at his desk. He would be expected to respond well to chiropractic care along with advice about setting up his workstation more suitably for his size.

Chapter summary

For each new patient that you see in clinic you will be required to assess their needs through careful questioning and examination in order to determine how best to manage their chiropractic care. You will be able to call upon the expertise of your clinic supervisor at all times but, as you gain experience, you will become more self-directed in your patient management and continue on your way to becoming a fully-fledged, reflective, patient-centred chiropractor.

Key points

- Chiropractic is practical, so you will practise your palpation and adjusting skills throughout the programme.

- During your studies you will be required to observe chiropractors and other healthcare professionals in practice.

- Self-reflection will form an important part of your development as a *thinking* practitioner.

- In your final clinical year, you will be responsible for the safe and ethical management of your own patient caseload (under supervision).

- Your final year caseload will amount to around 40 new patients.

- The last year will be the pinnacle of your chiropractic training – it is where the learning really begins!

Useful resources

Anglo-European College of Chiropractic: www.aecc.ac.uk

British Chiropractic Association:
www.chiropractic-uk.co.uk/For-You-77-Treatment-0-ms.aspx

McTimoney Chiropractic Association:
www.mctimoneychiropractic.org

McTimoney College of Chiropractic: www.mctimoney-college.ac.uk

University of Glamorgan, Faculty of Health, Sport and Science:
http://hesas.glam.ac.uk

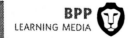

Chapter 12

Career progression after graduation

Rob Finch

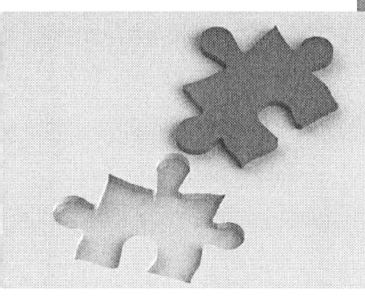

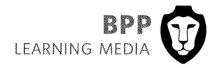

A career in chiropractic in the UK generally means working as a self-employed provider of private healthcare. Chiropractic care is rarely NHS-funded, so most patients either pay for their own treatment or are covered by private healthcare insurance. As a result, chiropractors often work in their own premises, although some provide their services in shared multidisciplinary clinics and work alongside other private healthcare practitioners, including podiatrists, physiotherapists and massage therapists. The careers of most chiropractors have a general clinical focus and follow a similar path. However, some practitioners develop their careers in a way that allows them to focus on particular patient groups, to undertake research, to teach others or to become involved in developing what is still a comparatively young profession. This chapter provides an overview of these exciting career pathways.

Competency and independence

Graduation from a chiropractic college represents an important step towards a career as an independent, primary-contact healthcare professional. A chiropractic qualification will enable you, as a graduate, to apply for registration with the General Chiropractic Council (GCC), which is the statutory regulator for the chiropractic profession in the UK. Registration with the GCC signals competence to practise and is a legal requirement.

The vast majority of UK-based chiropractors practise privately and your first job as a chiropractor is likely to be as an employed or self-employed associate in an established practice. Some graduates, particularly those who have had a previous career and experience of running a business, choose to set up their own practice immediately. However, the burden of securing finance, establishing premises and developing support structures (in addition to commencing independent clinical practice) means this is not a common option, nor one to be taken lightly (see Chapter 7). Many chiropractors, however, do eventually go on to open their own practice, perhaps in partnership with a colleague. This allows even greater independence in terms of shaping patient services and, for you, it could be the culmination of a long-term career aspiration.

Post-registration opportunities

Most healthcare professionals commence their career as a professional trainee, developing their initial clinical proficiency over a one- or two-year period by participating in a structured, vocational postgraduate training programme. In the UK, the chiropractic profession has developed such a programme known as Post-Registration Training (PRT), which is run by the College of Chiropractors (CoC). The PRT programme currently remains voluntary, but most chiropractors and chiropractic organisations recognise its importance, and successful completion is now a mandatory requirement for full membership of the main professional associations, or 'trade unions'. At some stage, it is possible that a vocational postgraduate training programme will become a statutory requirement – a necessity in terms of retaining statutory registration at the end of the first year of practice. In the meantime, responsible chiropractors participate in the voluntary programme noting that postgraduate training of this nature is the norm in medicine and other healthcare professions, and that it is rapidly becoming standard for chiropractic throughout Europe.

The College of Chiropractors is a postgraduate academic membership organisation with over 1,500 UK members and 2,800 members worldwide, with the following objectives:

- Promoting the art, science and practice of chiropractic
- Improving and maintaining standards in the practice of chiropractic for the benefit of the public
- Promoting awareness and understanding of chiropractic amongst medical practitioners and other healthcare professionals and the public
- Educating and training practitioners in the art, science and practice of chiropractic
- Advancing the study of and research in chiropractic (College of Chiropractors, 2005)

The CoC actively fosters patient and public partnership through a Lay Partnership Group (see Chapter 3). It offers members a wide and growing number of benefits, including bursaries for postgraduate study, a range of practice improvement tools and access to a UK-wide programme of subsidised Continuing Professional Development (CPD) events. The CPD events are run via a unique infrastructure of regional and expert groups or 'faculties'.

Post-registration training programme (PRT)

The PRT programme is run by the CoC. As a chiropractic graduate, it provides you with a structure for the first few months of your new career: setting requirements for the mentorship provided by the practice Principal, or other experienced chiropractor (known as the PRT

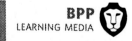

Trainer). As a PRT participant, you are also required to spend time observing other healthcare professionals. This provides mutual insight into respective clinical practices as well as helping to build referral relationships. Participants also spend time with their peers at regional PRT events and plan their future professional development by formally reflecting on their clinical experiences and the outcomes of their work. On successful completion of the PRT programme, you are eligible to take up Licentiate Membership of the CoC and full membership of your chosen professional association.

Formal postgraduate study

Some chiropractors choose to undertake formal postgraduate studies either immediately after qualification, or later on once their practice is established. A range of programmes are available at the undergraduate chiropractic colleges, but you could look to universities further afield and undertake master's courses on topics such as pain management, for example, or complementary therapies, including dry needling. You may want to specialise in particular areas of chiropractic (see Chapters 14 and 15). Passage through the levels of membership of the CoC is normally based on the achievement of postgraduate qualifications. Figure 12.1 indicates how different qualifications equate to the different membership levels. These levels are indicative of career progression.

The CoC also sets standards of practice in terms of meeting patient expectations and managing the clinical environment. It presents quality awards to recognise excellence in these areas. These awards, the Patient Partnership Quality Mark (PPQM) and the Clinical Management Quality Mark (CMQM), send out a strong message to patients and the public about the quality of chiropractic services in established clinics (See Chapter 3). The CoC accepts these quality marks as equivalents, in part, to postgraduate qualifications when awarding Membership and Fellowship.

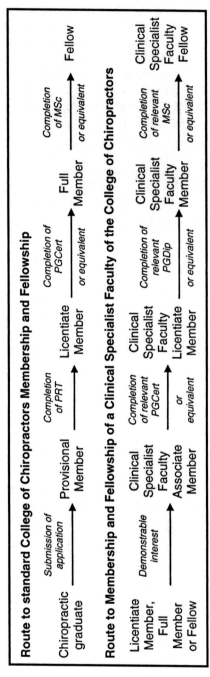

Figure 12.1: Career progression in the College of Chiropractors

Continuing Professional Development

Participation in the PRT programme helps satisfy many of the professional development needs of new graduates, but individuals start to recognise other developmental requirements as their careers progress, depending on personal preferences, strengths and weaknesses. Recognising individual aspirations and addressing them is an important component of your career development as a chiropractor and is addressed through a process known as Continuing Professional Development (CPD). Due to its perceived importance in ensuring practitioners remain up-to-date in their field, CPD is a statutory requirement; the GCC currently requires chiropractors to undertake at least 30 hours of self-directed learning each year, 15 hours of which must be undertaken with others.

Top tip

Continuing Professional Development is an important component of career development because the process involves identifying professional development needs and then planning and undertaking learning activities to address those needs.

As with many chiropractors, you might look to develop areas of special clinical interest, perhaps due to the particular patient population near your home, or due to your personal interests, such as sport. CPD provides a framework for developing your new skills and interests. Evaluating the learning activities planned and undertaken in these areas ensures a cyclical approach to career-based learning, and your interests can subsequently develop into a particular proficiency and ability to focus on specific patient groups.

Developing your career interests

In order to be recognised and referred to as a specialist in a particular field of practice, a healthcare practitioner's statutory regulator must have a specialist register which recognises areas of speciality and defines the competencies required to join it. The GCC does not currently have a specialist register, however some chiropractors do develop a career in which they are able to focus much of their professional activity on supporting and treating sportspeople, children or animals, for example.

Developing a special interest of this type usually follows from a period of intensive CPD, often in the form of a relevant postgraduate qualification, such as a PGCert (postgraduate certificate), PGDip (postgraduate diploma) or an MSc. A number of suitable postgraduate programmes are on offer, most of which can be followed on a part-time basis to allow candidates to continue clinical practice. Animal and paediatric chiropractic master's programmes, for example, are available as specialist post-graduate programmes. (see Chapter 6). Indeed, managing patients with needs relating to the field of study provides important learning material on which to reflect and gain relevant experience.

While there is no specialist register for chiropractors to join, the CoC recognises the additional knowledge, skills, experience and qualifications of chiropractors and awards Memberships and Fellowships of particular clinical specialist faculties. Members and Fellows of these faculties can look forward to exercising their skills under exciting circumstances, for example Sports Faculty members and Animal Faculty members can assist elite athletes (of the two- and four-legged variety, respectively) at major sporting events (see Chapter 15).

Case study: Paul Cheung

Paul Cheung became interested in sport and subsequently joined the CoC's Sports Faculty: 'I've been involved in professional football with Leeds United FC, Middlesbrough FC and Sheffield united FC. Also, I've had the privilege of working with my fellow international colleagues at the World Games in 2005, the Canoe-Polo World Championships in 2006, the British Masters Athletics and the Red Bull Formula 1 Team in 2007.'

Working in the NHS

Many chiropractors work alongside General Practitioners (GPs), and GPs often refer patients (particularly those with low back pain) to chiropractors (see Chapter 2). However, the vast majority of these patients are self-funded. Different approaches to healthcare commissioning over the years have resulted in sporadic purchasing of chiropractic services by the NHS so that it is unusual for patients to receive free chiropractic care at the point of delivery.

Opportunities exist for chiropractors to demonstrate their ability to offer high-quality musculoskeletal services by bidding for provider status but, as yet, it is uncertain whether significant numbers of chiropractors will be commissioned to provide NHS services in this way. Therefore, for the time being at least, you should consider a career in chiropractic as private and independent of government funding.

Teaching and training

Full-time and part-time undergraduate teaching positions are also available in the chiropractic educational institutions. Achievement of a relevant postgraduate master's degree is the normal minimum qualification for a full-time teaching position, although this is unlikely to be required for part-time technique or clinical teaching posts.

As a chiropractor with three or more years of postgraduate clinical experience, particularly if you are expanding your own practice, you might take on the role of PRT Trainer. Trainers provide the essential mentorship to support new chiropractors in their first months of practice and offer an opportunity to develop an interest in vocational training. You may find these roles of particular interest if you want a full-time clinical career but enjoy passing on your skills and providing guidance to less-experienced colleagues. This facilitates the professional development of others as well as yourself.

> 'I have been a regional tutor for several years, and taking time out from my busy clinic and other duties to nurture new graduates is difficult, but it always pays dividends. Their enthusiasm is inspiring. Being a PRT Trainer is a wonderful distraction from day-to-day clinic work, and if you have good teaching and communication skills, I highly recommend it.'

Research as a career option

An essential component of undergraduate training in chiropractic is the completion of a research project, which is written up as a detailed dissertation. While such a project is primarily an educational exercise, it may be the start of a long-term interest in research or even a distinct career choice for you. It is reasonably common for chiropractors to participate in research projects orchestrated by the academic institutions, or to design and conduct their own small-scale, clinic-based research. Private bursaries are available to enable chiropractors to undertake distance learning in advanced research methods to facilitate this activity, and some go on to undertake part-time research degrees, for example PhD or DChiro. It is less common for chiropractors to step back from clinical practice in order to undertake full-time research study but opportunities do exist, most notably within the educational institutions, if you are committed to a research career.

Shaping the profession

In the UK, the chiropractic profession is small but it has a complex structure. Not only does it have a dedicated regulator, it currently has four professional associations, a postgraduate professional membership college and three educational institutions providing undergraduate and postgraduate degree programmes. Additionally, there are numerous training organisations focusing on CPD provision in special interest areas and an independent Chiropractic Patients' Association. As a result, there are many ways for you to get involved in shaping the profession by taking on organisational and governance roles, and many chiropractors take an active and long-term interest in such activities.

Chapter summary

Chiropractic is a relatively young and small profession in the UK. This means that genuine and exciting opportunities exist for energetic graduates to develop a fulfilling and diverse career path: potentially combining effective clinical practice, running a successful business, teaching, participating in research and generally taking an active part in developing the profession.

Key points

- As a new chiropractic graduate, you must apply for registration with the GCC.

- You have to complete at least 30 hours of CPD every year to retain your registration.

- Most new graduates join the PRT programme during their first year in practice.

- There is a choice of professional associations to join which will support you.

- Post-graduate training allows you to develop specialist interests, such as treating animals or sportspeople.

- Once you have some experience, there is scope to teach or train other chiropractors.

- You can take part in research work via the CoC or conduct your own clinic-based projects.

Useful resources

Chiropractic Patients' Association: www.chiropatients.org.uk

College of Chiropractors: www.colchiro.org.uk

General Chiropractic Council: www.gcc-uk.org

References

College of Chiropractors (2005) *A Brief History of the College.* [Online] Available at: www.colchiro.org.uk/default.aspx?m=18mi=288 [Accessed 29 July 2012].

Chapter 13

Entering practice – what can you expect?

Matthew Bennett

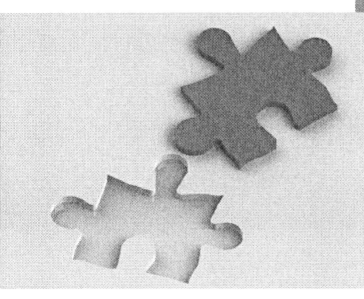

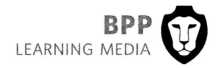

Your [first day in practice] is a bit like the first time you drive a car by yourself. You have had the training, the theory has been passed and you have done some supervised practical application, but it is the first time that you are alone and responsible for all the decisions you make.

Your first patient experience

Your first patient (say, Mrs Jones) walks into your treatment room, sits down and starts explaining her problem: a nasty low back pain that came on a couple of weeks ago. You listen intently as the occasional butterfly churns in your stomach. As you take more details of Mrs Jones's history, you start formulating the possible diagnoses which will point you towards the sort of tests and perhaps imaging, such as X-rays or MRIs, that you need to carry out or order.

Moving onto the examination, you run through the battery of orthopaedic and neurological tests that help rule out a serious disease and ultimately bring you to a probable diagnosis. Still, at the back of your mind you are wondering if you have missed anything. This patient might have a potentially life-threatening or crippling condition that needs urgent referral back to her GP. This is decision time! You have always had a tutor to point you in the right direction up until now, but here you are staring intently at your examination notes hoping the pertinent piece of information will jump out at you.

Finally, you decide you can help and you explain to Mrs Jones what you think is causing her back pain and proceed to outline a series of treatment visits during which you will carry out specific adjustments to the spinal joints that you think may be giving her trouble. You explain that you will be giving her some exercises to do and talking with her about lifestyle modifications at work and at home to help ease the discomfort and prevent recurrence. Mrs Jones gives her consent for treatment to start and you administer the first adjustment. As sometimes happens, her back pain is still there after you have finished adjusting, even though you explained that it would take several visits to achieve relief. In the end, Mrs Jones is reassured by your calm confidence (if only she knew!) and she makes her way home, knowing that you will call her that evening to make sure all is well.

Case study

Mr A, a 69-year-old accountant, had an appointment with a newly qualified chiropractor (on the recommendation of a colleague on leave) for a six-weekly general maintenance check. Just as the treatment finished the patient remarked, 'Oh, by the way, my calf hurts, perhaps I've pulled a muscle playing tennis'. On further examination, the new recruit found Mr A's right calf to be swollen and red, with the superficial veins prominent. It also felt warm compared to his left calf. The new chiropractor took the initiative, erring on the side of caution. He diagnosed a deep vein thrombosis (DVT) and advised Mr A to go straight to his GP. In fact, Mr A had been due to fly to Cyprus for a short family holiday that evening, which could have proved fatal with a DVT. Instead he was relaxing in the local hospital DVT unit, happy to be alive.

One job, many roles

That typical encounter with Mrs Jones tested several qualities that you will need as a clinician. You need to be a good communicator, which is more about listening than it is about talking. You have to be calm, confident and authoritative; safe in the knowledge that you are competent in your field. You will need empathy and a deep commitment to helping your patients. You will also need the manual dexterity in order to carry out sensitive palpation (hands-on examination) of the spine and other joints and tissues, as well as the physical fitness to be on your feet for large parts of the day – often carrying out manual treatment.

'At the end of my first week in practice I was so stiff and achy that I needed chiropractic care more than my patients did.' **Newly-qualified chiropractor**

You will need the depth of knowledge to carry out a detailed examination and arrive at an informed diagnosis and you will have to formulate a detailed plan of care, balanced with the patient's preferences. Then you will be required to carry out an effective treatment: all this while adhering to the General Chiropractic Council's (GCC's) *Code of Practice and Standard of Proficiency* (see Chapter 2), which requires certain standards to be met in practice.

One factor that attracts many to a chiropractic career is that it is not just about clinical work. The opportunities to run your own business mean that chiropractors often find their day-to-day activities can be quite varied. For instance, a typical chiropractor running their own clinic may work 80% of the time with patients, but spend the rest of the working week attending to accounts, marketing, staff management, clinic maintenance and DIY, as well as attending further postgraduate education courses and conferences.

> It is not just the clinical demands that will test you as a newly qualified chiropractor. You also might have to work as part of a team within a clinic and liaise with other professionals in your area. This not only includes General Practitioners (GPs) and consultants, but also other chiropractors, osteopaths and physiotherapists. You will also have to interact with employers or family members while maintaining patient confidentiality and other ethical boundaries (see Useful resources). You may come across hostile or sceptical attitudes by those who are unfamiliar with chiropractic and you will need to deal with these professionally and confidently.

Calling all entrepreneurs

Running your own business means that you may have to develop skills such as website design, newsletter writing, designing advertisements for a local newspaper or a poster for your reception area. You may choose to give talks to local community groups, in which case you may need to hone your public speaking skills. These are all things that you will either bring with you to practice or that you may need to learn after graduating.

You will be responsible for managing your own time. While there are certainly more demands if you are running your own clinic, there will still be jobs besides treating patients, even if you work in an established clinic. You will probably be responsible for your own tax accounts and have to submit a tax return if you are self-employed. Reports and letters will need to be written about patients, and clinical audits will be required to help measure and improve your performance. You may have telephone or email enquiries from patients or prospective patients asking you for your opinion or reassurance on various issues. Sometimes these responses can be urgent and will eat into a lunchtime break or keep you at work after hours, but it is your own business so you will want to put in this extra time to make it work.

Managing your caseload

One of the key demands of being a chiropractor is dealing with a full caseload while keeping to time. You will be able to decide how you choose to work: chiropractors see patients at different frequencies and intervals, some for ten-minute sessions more frequently, for example, and some for half-hour sessions less frequently. If you are to keep to your appointment times, you will need to work quickly and methodically while maintaining concentration without becoming brusque or distant. If you run over time with a just few patients you can quite easily run substantially behind, leaving patients waiting in reception becoming more and more irritated. If you have an urgent call to return at the same time and you need the toilet, it may take a certain character to maintain equanimity! Learning how to manage a full caseload, on time and with poise, is something you will be prepared for during your clinical training in college.

A lifetime of learning

As in other healthcare professions, graduation is just the first step in a lifetime of learning. After several years of hard work at a chiropractic college it is liberating to be freed from formal learning and regular exams. Many chiropractors, however, go on to study areas of special interest, such as sports chiropractic, animal chiropractic, paediatrics, specialist techniques or imaging. A few graduates continue to a further postgraduate degree, making them eligible for Fellowship of the College of Chiropractors (CoC). (See Chapter 12). As a chiropractor you are also required to submit an annual Continuing Professional Development report to the General Chiropractic Council (GCC), which outlines the postgraduate training you have done over the previous year and which is required for continuing registration to practise.

Your first decision

Before you even start in practice you will have some big decisions to make. Do you want to work for someone else in an established practice or work by yourself by either starting or buying your own practice? The advantages of working for someone else are that you often get more support, you may have an existing patient list to take over and you do not have the hassle of running your own business. On the other hand, working independently has many attractions: you can determine the type of practice you want to run and the sort of caseload you want to attract as well as choosing your own staff, for instance.

Whatever decision you make about the way you want to set up your practice, you will be supported by the CoC, which runs a scheme for new graduates. The CoC promotes professional excellence for postgraduates by running courses and seminars, promoting research and providing pathways for professional progression through associateship, membership and then fellowship. The first step on this path is the CoC's Post-Registration Training (PRT) scheme (see Chapter 12).

College of Chiropractors Post-Registration Training

The CoC's PRT scheme partners you with a clinical trainer who supports you in the transition between clinical work as a student to that of a fully-fledged chiropractor. A trainer will observe you intermittently through your first year and allow you opportunities to observe them. They will offer feedback and advice, and generally help you develop your skills, and answer your questions. There are also seminars where you get together with other new graduates and a tutor to discuss everything from patient management to dealing with emergencies and running your own business.

Your professional life and responsibilities do not stop when you close the door of your clinic at the end of a hard day. Certain standards of behaviour outside work are important in all professions. You are likely to live and work in the same community as your patients and their friends and relatives. If you have been practising in a town for a while, you are likely to bump into patients in the street or in the pub. At first this can be a bit disconcerting, but you may find that this is outweighed by the esteem and respect that people give you in response to your professional status.

Top tip

You can get support from one of the professional associations (see Useful resources). These organisations provide services, such as medical malpractice insurance, advice on setting up and running a business, employment contract templates and conflict resolution, as well as regular conferences. They also provide lobbying power so that your voice is heard where it matters.

Your future in chiropractic

There will undoubtedly be some interesting opportunities within chiropractic over the next few years. At present there is limited access for patients wanting to use chiropractic on the NHS. This may well change in due course and currently chiropractors may work alongside doctors and physiotherapists in hospitals and General Practitioner surgeries, as well as accepting NHS patients in their private practice in much the same way as a dentist might. More and more sports teams are using chiropractors as part of their medical staff and opportunities at sports competitions continue to improve. New research shows that chiropractic care can be effective, not only in the treatment of musculoskeletal injuries, but also in injury prevention and performance enhancement and it is likely that chiropractors will become more commonplace in professional and amateur sports.

A package of care

Chiropractic is often described as offering a package of care rather than providing a stand-alone treatment. Indeed, the scope of chiropractic practice is very broad. Besides the core manual therapy skills that you develop, you may choose further training: for example, in nutrition to help patients with supplements and diet; acupuncture to help with pain control and muscle relaxation or neurology to help with reading, learning and behavioural problems. It may be that practising full-time does not appeal to you. There are many other opportunities within chiropractic, including research, teaching and contributing to the development of the profession through the professional committee structures. As the chiropractic profession is relatively small, the opportunities for new graduates are perhaps greater in these areas than in the larger professions.

Chapter summary

First and foremost, patients are at the heart of chiropractic practice. When your skills have helped an elderly woman to walk to the shops and back, a sportsman get that extra second in performance, or someone in danger of losing their job to get back to work, you will realise what a truly satisfying vocation chiropractic can be.

Your first patient encounter – alone and officially unsupervised – will be testing – but remember, you have the training and the skills to see it through. The college exit exams are rigorous and you will not have graduated if you are not up to the job. You should feel nervous – if you start to feel complacent about your work as a chiropractor, alarm bells should ring. The extra adrenaline that your first cases (and later on, difficult cases) induce will keep you attuned to your patient's needs – some of which will not be straight forward.

Key points

- Your life as a chiropractor will be varied and rewarding.
- You will need good communication skills in addition to clinical training.
- Chiropractic practice can be physically demanding.
- Good business and administration skills are important.
- You can expect support from professional bodies.
- A commitment to lifelong learning is important.

Useful resources

British Chiropractic Association: www.chiropractic-uk.co.uk

GCC *Code of Practice and Standard of Proficiency*: www.gcc-uk.org/page.cfm?page_id=15

McTimoney Chiropractic Association: www.mctimoneychiropractic.org

Post registration training scheme: www.colchiro.org.uk/default.aspx?m=3&mi=173

Scottish Chiropractic Association: www.sca-chiropractic.org

United Chiropractic Association: www.united-chiropractic.org

Chapter 14

Insights into specialist practice – animals

Marisa Pinnock

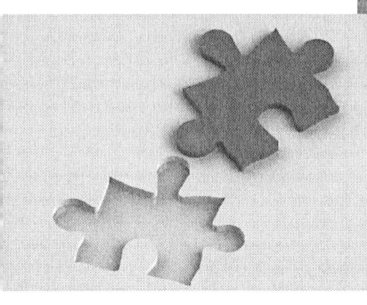

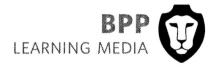

Many people who love animals believe it would be a dream job to spend every day with them making them feel better and knowing the animal is thankful to their 'saviour' for the chiropractic care that they have received. The reality is that you need to be prepared to spend long hours outside in pouring rain, freezing cold and driving wind. You can spend hours driving from one location to another in traffic jams with poor directions only to find that the owners are not there when you arrive. However, on those marvellous warm, sunny days when you are in the most beautiful spot in the country and you have just treated an animal that has been in pain and you see an obvious change (the animal shakes itself and looks at you so gratefully), you find a balance and know you have a truly rewarding vocation.

Animals can be perfect patients

Animals are very sensitive to chiropractic care and you can often see amazing results. All chiropractors who adjust animals can recount stories of miraculous turnarounds: saving animals destined to be put to sleep or changing the lives of animals that have been in pain or had a restricted lifestyle, sometimes for years. If you like working outside, love animals and have the skill to handle them confidently and safely, animal chiropractic has to be one of the most rewarding professions in the world.

Animals in general are very responsive to chiropractic, partly because they behave as they are supposed to behave, as four-legged animals! Typically, an initial course of chiropractic for people may be between three to six sessions but animals tend to need fewer as they are 'in tune' with what their body needs. This is unlike human beings, who may spend many hours hunched over laptops, driving cars or slouching on couches after seeing their own chiropractor.

What are the legalities?

The Veterinary Surgeons Act of 1966 controls the care of animals in the UK. The main aim of the Act is to prevent laypeople from practising 'veterinary surgery', so the primary care of every animal must be under the supervision of a veterinary surgeon (vet) to ensure the safety of the animal. There are exceptions, however, and chiropractic for animals is covered under the Exemption Order of 1962 which counts as a manipulative therapy in this context. You will still need to get permission from a veterinary surgeon (vet) if you are going to adjust an animal, but chiropractic is very well recognised as an important and effective intervention for animal musculoskeletal health.

As an animal chiropractor you are also governed by the General Chiropractic Council (GCC), which is the statutory body responsible for regulating chiropractic under the Chiropractors Act of 1994. In effect, you will have two legal acts to adhere to. (See Useful resources.)

Teamwork is key

When treating animals, you have to be prepared to work within a team. The vet is the critical starting point. Vets are the people who can refer an animal to you for chiropractic, so it is crucial that you build up good relationships with the vets in your area so that they know what you can do, how well educated you are and what cases you can help them with. As a chiropractor, often the most effective way of teaching vets what you do and the results you can achieve is to treat them personally. When you are in practice, you should report back to them what you have found and, very importantly, you should refer back to them if it there is something outside your scope of practice that needs veterinary intervention. Just as chiropractors have an obligation to refer their human patients back to the medical profession if they feel a case is more appropriate for them to deal with so with their animal patients, the obligation is to refer back to the vet.

Equine chiropractic

If you are interested in working with horses then the team will start to grow larger as you will need to involve the blacksmith to check the foot balance of the horse, the saddler to make sure the tack is fitting properly, the dentist to make sure there are no problems in the mouth and, quite often, the trainer of the horse. Do not forget that it is quite common to find that the rider is sitting incorrectly or that riding methods have led to the horse's pain. Tact and diplomacy may well be needed to balance all the egos of the team concerned with the horse's welfare. You will need a good background of knowledge in all these areas to identify the problem and suggest changes that will help the horse without upsetting any individuals.

Why would a horse need chiropractic?

Horses require chiropractic for much the same reasons as humans require it:

- Acute injury after accidents and trauma
- Maintenance of the body as it gets older
- Care of a body that is already compromised by shape, injury, training methods or poor riding
- Treatment of undiagnosed problems after thorough veterinary examination

The principle indications for equine chiropractic evaluation are back or neck pain, localised or regional joint stiffness, poor performance, or an altered gait that may or may not be associated with lameness. Initially, a thorough case history and diagnostic examination by the vet are necessary to identify soft tissue and osseous (bone) pathology, neurological or nerve disorders or other lameness conditions that may not be responsive to chiropractic care. Once the vet has asked the chiropractor to examine the horse, manual palpation and gait evaluation (looking to see how the horse moves) are used to localise and identify soft tissue and osseous structures for changes in texture, tissue mobility, or resistance to pressure.

Trained equine chiropractors should be able to evaluate vertebral (spinal) disorders and determine if a horse's back problem, for example, will be potentially responsive to chiropractic care or if the condition should have further diagnostic evaluation or be better managed with traditional veterinary care.

Indications for chiropractic evaluation of horses

- Changes in behaviour, including avoidance (either while ridden or on the ground)
- Poor performance
- Back or neck pain, or reduced neck or back flexibility
- Localised muscle tightness
- Vague lameness, or lame only when ridden
- Uneven or asymmetric gait
- Recent changes in body shape / spinal curve
- Difficult or improper saddle fit
- Discomfort with saddle placement or mounting
- Horse resents tightening of the girth

- Stiff and slow to warm up
- Bucks or lays ears back when ridden
- Constantly on one rein or line
- Difficulty with a lead or gait transition
- Refusal of jumps or resisting collection
- Tilting of the head or difficulty turning in one direction
- Consistently stumbling or dragging a toe
- Muscle mass or pelvic asymmetry
- Inability to stand squarely on all four limbs
- Difficulty standing for the farrier
- Holds tail to one side or resents being groomed.

An equine chiropractor is often now a valued member of a team looking after top competition horses and can be seen at supporting many disciplines, including three-day eventers, show jumpers, dressage competitors, combined driving participants, endurance riders and horse racers.

Other creatures, great and small

Horses are not the only animals that benefit from chiropractic – pretty much any animal that has a spine can, in theory, benefit, but for practical reasons (and sometimes for the safety of the chiropractor if the animal is large or dangerous) some species are seen very rarely. Many farm animals live in situations that can give rise to problems: cows, for instance, can 'do the splits' with their hind legs on slippery concrete and sheep may have problems in lambing (as might the lambs that are pulled out of them). Unfortunately, regardless of whether or not chiropractic can help, and usually for financial reasons, the chiropractor is only called if the animal is a high-quality show or stud animal, or if they are a pet or of sentimental value.

Obviously, if you or your friends or family own farm animals, then your help can be enlisted if the vet is in agreement. This is when you can spend hours in the cold, wet slurry fighting with a beast in pain that has no idea you are trying to help it. But the benefit that you can bring will outweigh that personal discomfort in the end. Interestingly, some zoos, safari parks and petting farms have regular visits by chiropractors to check the health of their animals: this is more often the case if they have a vet who uses a chiropractor as part of their veterinary team.

Case study

'My own experience is varied: I have treated orphan lambs kept in the warming oven of an Aga, geese with damaged necks from fox attacks, goats that have fallen down cliffs and I have given health checks to many species of zoo animals, including alpacas, lemurs and even elephants! (All great fun to relate at dinner parties, but much more meaningful when you see the results.) An avian vet once referred a Chinese goose to me that he had diagnosed with sciatica. The female goose had not stood up for over a week (following overzealous behaviour by her mate), she was not eating and was quite poorly and the gander was beside himself fussing over her. I assessed her and made an adjustment to her pelvis following which she stood up, shook herself and walked off eating grass. I do not know who was most amazed – the goose, the gander, the owner or myself!'

Chiropractic for small animals

In private practice you can see a range of species kept as pets. Many dog owners seek chiropractic, but so do owners of cats, poultry, rabbits and other small mammals. Cats are very good at looking after themselves and, generally, you would only see a cat that had been involved in an accident (often hit by a car) once the vet has decided that any fractures or other damage are stable. It can be several years after the accident that a cat is first presented, but the full case history often elicits the explanation that the cat 'has never been the same since...'. After chiropractic, the owner will be delighted that to have their 'old cat back' and the cat is much happier as well. Owners who have regular chiropractic themselves may ask the vet whether they can bring their older cat for maintenance care and, as with other species, this can make a cat more comfortable.

Canine chiropractic – a range of opportunities

According to the latest figures presented by the PFMA (Pet Food Manufacturers' Association) there were approximately 8 million dogs owned as pets in the UK in 2012, which means that around 23% of the UK population own at least one dog. Many people keep dogs simply as pets or companions while others work dogs in many disciplines: working in trials, agility, flyball and obedience competitions or showing or shooting. Dogs also work professionally with the police, customs and excise, as guide dogs for the blind or hard of hearing and for security companies. As owners become educated about the benefits of chiropractic, having been looked after well themselves, they start to enquire about chiropractic for their dogs.

> 'I have found working with dogs so rewarding. Chiropractic helps dogs for exactly the same reasons that it helps horses, small animals or people: trauma, age, maintaining performance or assisting in diagnosis with difficult cases.'

Dogs can be involved in accidents quite often: running together as a pack or with friends involves bashing into each other: older dogs can be 'T-boned' by younger, more exuberant puppies, or accidents can happen in their working life, perhaps hitting a jump, falling down a ditch or just slipping on bad ground. Once the vet has referred the dog, the chiropractor will go through the same routine of assessment as with a horse before deciding that chiropractic is indicated.

Many professionals who work with dogs have realised that chiropractic is a cost-effective way to keep a dog performing at maximum efficiency. Professional dogs can cost a huge amount of money to train: to search for drugs and assist the police, for example, or to make a blind person's life more normal. Everyone relies on these dogs to do their best under all conditions and it can be in a dog's nature to work regardless of discomfort. A good handler may recognise when a dog's behaviour has changed, even subtly, and they may also see the difference that chiropractic makes. Institutions and companies might then make a policy that their working dogs are checked once or twice a year to keep them performing at their best. Owners of competition dogs are also very observant when their dogs start slowing down in the weaves, even by a second or so. They also find that a chiropractic check up every few months can knock several seconds off their dog's time.

Case study

Molly was a five-year-old yellow Labrador retriever. She was a healthy, very lively bitch who was not overweight and has had no previous visits to the vet apart from annual check ups and vaccinations. A year ago she became intermittently lame on her right forelimb. She was taken to the vet, who advised rest and anti-inflammatory medication. This did not help, so she was given a general anaesthetic and her shoulder, elbow and front leg were

BPP
LEARNING MEDIA

X-rayed. Nothing abnormal was found, but the intermittent lameness continued. Chiropractic was suggested on a recommendation from a friend. The vet agreed and Molly presented for treatment. The history taking revealed that she always slept with her head propped on something; a wall or a cushion at a very odd angle. Physical examination showed that the vertebrae in her neck were rotated and these were adjusted. Molly's owners remembered that, at ten months, Molly ran head long into a moving car. No further treatment was given initially, but when Molly returned for the second visit her owners were thrilled that she had been sound for much of the time. After three visits, her neck was completely better and she was totally recovered.

Top tip

Animals perform at their best when all their joints are functioning as well as they can regardless of age. This is why chiropractic can play an important part in the life of any animal, especially a competition animal since it is, essentially, an athlete.

How will I practise as an animal chiropractor?

It will depend on you and how much you want to work with animals and also whether you like working with horses or dogs, or both. Some chiropractors will only have an animal practice, but the majority split their time between days in the clinic treating people and days on the road treating horses. Generally the chiropractor will visit a horse in its natural surroundings which can mean that you spend a lot of time driving between locations. It is therefore much better if you can get an agreement with a local stable or yard so that you see multiple horses at each visit. With dogs it is slightly different. Generally dogs will be brought to your clinic location and so your time can be spent much more cost-effectively as there is no travelling time to be factored in. But remember, you will need a completely separate dog clinic as you cannot see animals and people in the same physical location for obvious health and safety reasons.

How do I train as an animal chiropractor?

There are a number of continuing professional development courses available in the UK that will teach you skills in how to adjust animals, but currently there is only one master's level programme available: the MSc Animal Manipulation, run by the McTimoney College of Chiropractic (MCC) (see Chapter 6). Graduates of this programme are very well respected by vets and owners alike and you will be entitled to become a Fellow of the Specialist Faculty of Animal Chiropractic of the College of Chiropractors (see Chapter 12). You can enrol on this two-year part-time programme as soon as you graduate as a chiropractor, and you will be taught all the necessary scientific and clinical skills in order to build your animal practice.

BPP LEARNING MEDIA

Chapter summary

Chiropractic is extremely well received by animals on the whole, and few object to care unless they are in a lot of pain or have had bad experiences in other hands. Many animals that are treated regularly show that they are expecting a good experience: dogs pull to get into the treatment room and greet the chiropractor very exuberantly, horses stand quietly and show they are enjoying what is being done by licking, chewing, lowering their head and obviously relaxing. The owners can see the obvious enjoyment and benefits that the animal has after chiropractic and often then book in with a chiropractor themselves. They understand that the animal cannot be experiencing a 'placebo' effect and sometimes seeing such dramatic changes makes them realise that chiropractic works! As such, chiropractic for animals is a fantastic advertisement for the profession as a whole.

Key points

- Animal chiropractic can be challenging, but when you see obvious changes the rewards are great.

- Animals can be amazingly sensitive to chiropractic, which defies the placebo effect.

- When working with animals, you will need to abide by the Veterinary Surgeons Act as well as the Chiropractors Act.

- You should be prepared to work in a team (including vets, owners, trainers and saddlers etc).

- Horses, dogs, cats and other animals can benefit from chiropractic care.

Useful resources

College of Chiropractors: www.colchiro.org.uk

MSc Animal Manipulation:
www.mctimoney-college.ac.uk/courses-cpd/msc-animal-manipulation

MSc Chiropractic Small Animals course: www.mctimoney-college.ac.uk/courses-cpd/msc-chiropractic-small-animals

Royal College of Veterinary Surgeons: www.rcvs.org.uk/home

Reference

PFMA (Pet Food Manufacturers' Association) (2012) *Annual Report 2012* [online] Available at: www.pfma.org.uk/pfma-annual-report-2012/ [Accessed 9 January 2013].

Chapter 15

Insights into specialist practice – sports

Richard Skippings

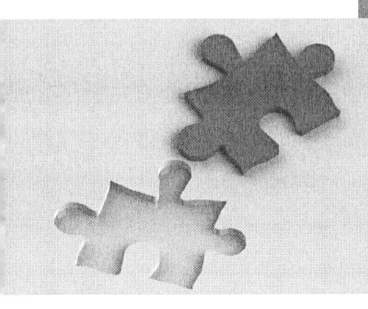

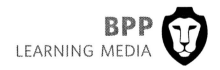

Once you have graduated as a chiropractor, you will be competent in general practice, knowing a little about a lot of things. When you have been in practice for a while you may well develop an interest in a specialist area, as happens in the rest of the medical world. You may wish to remain in general practice and develop general skills or you may find that there are certain groups of people whom you enjoy treating the most. You may also have particular interests of your own that push you towards a specialist field of work.

You will inevitably want to improve your knowledge and expertise in a chosen field with further postgraduate education and qualifications. In order to retain your registration with the General Chiropractic Council (GCC), you have to do a certain amount of Continuing Professional Development (CPD) and it is logical to document your postgraduate education in your personal chosen field to fulfil this legal requirement (see Chapters 2 and 12). In the UK, the College of Chiropractors (CoC) Specialist Clinical Faculty for Sport and Exercise acts as a conduit for this kind of postgraduate education, providing seminars on specific sports topics and mentoring at sports events.

Top tip

Progression through the CoC membership categories in the Faculty for Sport and Exercise demonstrates a higher level of expertise and knowledge compared with the general practice chiropractor.

Sport and exercise medicine – a growing field

In the last 20 years, the field of sports injury management has enjoyed ever-increasing recognition as a subspecialty within the healthcare professions, culminating in the recent elevation of 'sport and exercise medicine' as a specialty within the NHS. During this time there have also been huge advances in our understanding of how injuries occur, how to treat them, manage their recovery, return to activity and help prevent injuries in the first place. The UK government and other health bodies have also tried to encourage people to take more regular exercise in order to improve general health. Regular exercise has been shown to impart health benefits, particularly the reduced likelihood of heart disease, type II diabetes and depression, and it also gives an increased feeling of wellbeing. As a result of this and other initiatives, people have become much more health conscious and the numbers involved in sport and exercise have proliferated.

This means an increase in sport- and exercise-related injuries and conditions for which people seek treatment. Injuries that occur in sport and exercise are, generally, the same as those that happen in everyday life. They are, however, more likely to occur during sport and exercise, and may be more serious because of the increased loads that are placed on the body due to the higher intensity of activity experienced.

Case study

A 42-year-old local club cricketer presented with a stiff and painful shoulder and neck. This had started after winter net practice and was diagnosed as an overuse injury straining the muscles of the shoulder girdle that affected the function of the neck. The problems were caused by too much bowling during a two-hour session while not being fit enough to sustain that level of activity. The patient had had a four-month break from the end of the season to the start of net practice so he had lost all cricket conditioning – no surprise, therefore, that he had symptoms. A course of treatment together with a rehabilitation programme and a pre-season fitness programme were necessary to help prevent a recurrence in subsequent years.

How can I get involved in sports chiropractic?

If you choose to be involved in this field of work, there are a number of different ways in which you can work in sports chiropractic. Some chiropractors choose (and are lucky enough) to work with sports teams or clubs. Many professional teams employ the services of chiropractors to support their athletes; these teams include football teams, rugby, formula 1 racing, cycling and others. Chiropractors can work with organisations and provide treatment services at sporting events for all participants. Recently, events in the UK that have involved chiropractors include golf, athletics championships, rugby tournaments, tug-of-war championships, clay pigeon shooting championships and hockey tournaments. These events can be at a local level, which is a good place to start and to gain experience up to national and international level.

"I've been a rugby fanatic since primary school and played at a high amateur level until my early twenties when I injured my knee badly during a tackle. Luckily, my club at the time had an arrangement with a local chiropractor who had me playing again within weeks. When I became disenchanted with my job as a salesman, I decided to study chiropractic so I could stay involved in the game and provide similar support to young players. It's a decision I don't regret!" **Member of the College of Chiropractors Faculty for Sport and Exercise.**

What challenges might I face?

Working at events or matches will certainly mean that you see a lot more acute injuries, which require immediate assessment and treatment. This requires the skills, expertise and knowledge to work quickly and efficiently to determine the severity of the injury and whether or not the player can continue to play or be withdrawn.

Top tip

A detailed knowledge of a particular sport is vital when you attend to acute sporting injuries so that you have an understanding of the mechanisms of injury.

As a 'sports chiropractor', you may choose to work solely in a clinical setting in which an athlete attends your clinic for chiropractic. This will give you more time to formulate a course of care that would include a rehabilitation programme and a plan for a return to activity and competition. This can be achieved, in cooperation with the athlete's support team (coaches and trainers etc), to provide the best long-term support for the athlete. It also gives you the time and opportunity to develop rehabilitation programmes to help with injury avoidance and to provide periodical monitoring and assessment of the fitness state of the athlete (which would be carried out in conjunction with the sports specialists attached to clubs or individuals).

In your regular clinic you will also see many patients who play sports for recreational reasons and those who exercise to be fit and healthy but do not choose to compete. These people may also need the attention of a chiropractor who specialises in sport and exercise. In such cases, where the patient does not have access to the sports medicine and sports science teams of the elite, the chiropractor will be administering a complete package of care. This means that, as well as assessment, diagnosis and treatment of the sporting injury, as a chiropractor with special sports training, you will be managing the rehabilitation and return-to-play programme as well.

Case study: Modern pentathlons

A promising 12-year-old modern pentathlete presented with anterior (frontal) lower leg and low back pain that had started after a cross-country run in heavy mud one week earlier. This was aggravated by running and was affecting her training. Mechanical joint dysfunction was identified in the low back and pelvis, which caused a lower limb imbalance that stressed the muscles of the lower leg. Her running style was also analysed and showed that she was wearing the wrong type of shoes; the effects of which were exaggerated by running on heavy ground precipitating the injury. Treatment of the injury and a rehabilitation programme resolved the problem and obtaining the correct footwear helped to prevent any recurrences.

Maintenance is key

When dealing with athletes as a chiropractor, you will sometimes see athletes who are fit. These people have nothing wrong with them (as far as they are aware). They will come to see you because they know that you understand the mechanics of the body and that, in order for them to perform to their maximum potential, they must be functioning correctly. They will be looking for injury prevention and performance enhancement (anything to give them an edge over their competitors), as part of their pre- and post-competition routine and to help them maintain form.

At other times the subject will be an athlete who is already carrying old injuries or who has recurring injuries. This will often happen at championships where an athlete is injured, but simply *has* to compete. They will often be looking for a 'quick fix' to get them through and, hopefully, to perform better. If you do find a mechanical problem in such a case, it might be a mistake to correct it immediately prior to their event. Changing something significant, especially before a technical event, might upset an athlete's rhythm and cause a decrease in performance. If this is the case, the best thing to do is get them through the event and then invite them back for more work when you both have more time before the next event. You may also be asked to deal with emergencies when an athlete has an acute injury. This could be something simple, like 'going over on an ankle' in a warm up or a more serious case, such as a neck or head injury, which requires referral and may often present if you are working pitch-side for a team involved in a contact sport like rugby.

Case study

Two British chiropractors, Jesper Dahl and Ian Dingwall, work regularly on the European and the Professional Golfers Association of America tours with Pro-Golf Health, a multi-disciplinary sports health company. Both are certified golf medical practitioners qualified via the Titleist Performance Institute (another provider of sport-specific postgraduate education). After Charl Schwartzel won the US Masters at Augusta in 2011, Pro-Golf Health's clients included three out of the four major championship winners. The company's comprehensive programmes look at the professional golfer as a whole, implementing a wide range of therapeutic interventions and strategies. These include chiropractic, physiotherapy, massage, reflex and fascial therapies, cardiovascular fitness, core stability, flexibility, strength and conditioning training, as well as dietary and nutritional advice.

Postgraduate education

Top tip

Although there are other sports-related master's programmes available in the UK, at present there is no specific sports chiropractic master's degree you can enrol on post graduation. The following routes however will provide you with a focus to help you develop your sports-centred practice:

- The CoC Faculty for Sport & Exercise provides a forum for Continuing Professional Development (CPD) and post-graduate education.

- The CoC organises seminars, workshops and mentoring for those interested in developing their knowledge, skills and expertise in dealing with sports injuries.

- Progression through the membership categories demonstrates that you are keeping up-to-date with developments in the field and increasing your scope and depth of knowledge and expertise.

The CoC seminars are open to all those with an interest in sports chiropractic and can be taken as stand-alone events without the commitment to undertake a full course of training. Starting as a new graduate with an interest in sports, you can initially become a Licentiate Member and, finally, after becoming a full Member, you can progress to being a Specialist Fellow of the CoC as you increase your knowledge and skills. There are criteria you must fulfil at each stage, and at least five years of experience as a chiropractor and / or completion of a relevant masters degree will qualify you for the coveted status of Fellow of the Sports and Exercise Faculty.

Other chiropractic sports bodies

The British Chiropractic Sports Council (BCS) is an organisation of chiropractors who work at tournaments or championships and who are associated with clubs or sports organisations. This organisation is also affiliated with the Fédération Internationale de Chiropratique du Sport (FICS) and has access to their postgraduate study programme, the International Chiropractic Sports Science Diploma (ICSSD), which is recognised by the CoC as counting towards Licentiate membership. Many sports chiropractors are members of both organisations due to the different roles that they fulfil.

Chiropractic and the Olympics

At the 2010 winter Olympics in Vancouver, chiropractors were officially included for the first time in the history of the games. They gave treatments in the Olympic polyclinic, which the host nation provides to give medical support to the athletes and officials during the games. This arrangement was carried forward to the summer games in the 2012 London Olympics and Paralympics, when 30 chiropractors were involved in treating athletes, officials and others belonging the Olympic 'family'.

Tom Greenway (who has also worked in premiership football and with elite athletics) was the chiropractic lead on the physical therapies stream of the London Organising Committee of the Olympic and Paralympic Games (LOCOG). He spent six years negotiating the inclusion of chiropractors and how they were to be best utilised and where. The chiropractors involved worked in the three polyclinics located at the Olympic village for most sports and were part of a multidisciplinary team which included sports doctors, physiotherapists, massage therapists and osteopaths, providing the best possible care for the athletes giving appropriate and timely management of their conditions – everything that an athlete could possibly wish for! It is hoped that as part of the legacy of the 2012 Olympic games, this arrangement will become permanent so that chiropractors will be included in the future summer and winter games.

Chapter summary

Chiropractic is ideally suited to helping sportspeople achieve their potential – working, as it does, on the neuro-musculoskeletal system and impacting on general health. If you have a personal interest in sport, you can combine your passion with a fulfilling career as a chiropractor.

Key points

- A focus on sports chiropractic would suit the sports-minded chiropractic student.

- In practice, sports chiropractic offers a varied and challenging way of working.

- Postgraduate qualifications are essential if you want to progress in your career.

- This special interest presents the possibility of travelling with teams or organisations around the world.

- Working in a team with other healthcare professionals provides a very satisfying career environment.

Useful resources

College of Chiropractors Faculty Sport and Exercise Faculty: www.colchiro.org.uk/default.aspx?m=21&mi=139&ms=29&title=Spo rt%20&%20Exercise%20-

Fédération Internationale de Chiropratique du Sport: http://fics-sport.org

The British Chiropractic Sports Council: www.chirosport.org

Chapter 16

Research – developing the profession

'If we knew what it was we were doing, it would not be called research, would it?' (Albert Einstein)

Adrian Hunnisett

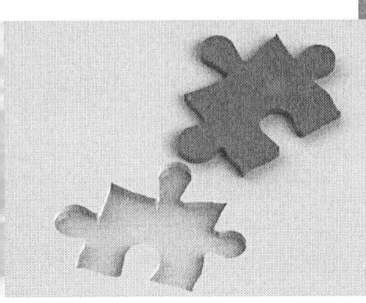

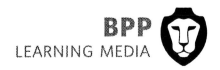

During the course of your chiropractic studies, you will come across the terms 'evidence', 'evidence-based practice', 'research', and 'dissertation' time and time again. As a student you will have to carry out some research during your programme of study. Usually, this is in the form of an individual project or dissertation during your final year of study. The preparation for this final work may take place over a number of semesters to get you ready for the challenges ahead. Many colleges and universities are now introducing elements of research-based or enquiry-based learning into all levels of study, giving students exposure to a research culture at an early stage. Initially you may be a bit scared about the thought of doing research, but once you have the satisfaction of completing your own project, and perhaps even getting it published, you will feel differently about it!

Why study research at chiropractic college?

The research elements of your programme are designed to provide you with a number of skills that will enhance your abilities to think and appraise critically. These skills help you to formulate questions about chiropractic practice, identify sources of existing data, collect and analyse new data and then formulate new theories and ideas. In the chiropractic profession, these skills will act as the basis for your Continuing Professional Development (CPD, see Chapter 12) and enhance your problem-solving abilities in your everyday work. In other words, 'What could I do differently to help patients better?' This is the start of professional lifelong learning.

The word 'research' invariably strikes a degree of terror into the hearts of some students, many of whom are not interested in research and have no experience of it. In addition, students may perceive research as difficult, time-consuming and, at undergraduate level, as not serving any useful purpose other than 'ticking an academic box'. The latter perception is entirely wrong and probably stems from a lack of understanding of what research actually is. The aim of this chapter is to demystify research and to show you how it can help you grow as a person through your studies and also raise the awareness of chiropractic.

What is research?

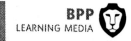

> **Definition:**
>
> Research (from the French verb, *rechercher*), means to 'seek out' and refers to the search for knowledge.

Broadly, research is about collecting and analysing data of various forms in a systematic way to enhance our understanding of a topic. This may involve establishing new facts or solving problems. The topic itself may not be anything new, but research may throw new light on a topic or analyse it from a new perspective.

This topic gives you the opportunity to pursue interests you have developed over the programme of your studies. It helps you to learn more about something new, to hone your problem-solving skills and to challenge yourself in new ways. It is at the heart of academic life and is one of the defining characteristics of higher education that differentiates it from other forms of training. In general, research falls into three main categories:

1. **Pure (or basic) research:** identifying new developments through systematic documentation, data collection and interpretation of a topic for the advancement of knowledge. This tends to lend itself more to laboratory-based work and relies on strict adherence to protocols.

2. **Applied research:** the research, methods and outcomes address specific workplace topics and deal with solving practical problems. It is therefore 'business-driven'. This discipline draws heavily on the findings of pure research to form a basis for enquiry and is certainly applicable to chiropractic.

3. **Action research:** deals with change management. This type of research plans to alter something and identifies the changes that result. The outcome of this type of research can significantly improve our understanding of the original problem, which may be chiropractic related.

Research in everyday life

Everyone does research, even your grandmother. She wants to buy you a Christmas present and knows you love woolly mittens (or you did when you were three!). Granny then looks in the telephone directory (against the advice of your mother) and makes a list of all the local shops that sell woollen mittens. She goes into town, looks at all the mittens, then asks the shop assistant about the price, thickness and how waterproof they are and so on. Using her new-found knowledge, she finds a pair at a price she is prepared to pay, purchases them, wraps them in Christmas paper and gives them to you on Christmas Day.

Your grandmother has undertaken research in order to purchase the correct type of mittens at the right price. Her research was very systematic; building on her existing knowledge and assessing the available options before moving forward. Whatever the research category, the key part is 'systematic enquiry', and a logical approach to research ensures that the value of the study is maintained and that your findings are valid.

What is evidence?

Essentially, evidence is defined as the data used to support a conclusion or theory. On detective television programmes, for example, you will be aware that the police generally have a suspicion of who has committed the crime (the theory). The programme then focuses on gathering material to prove, or disprove that theory (the evidence). The same principle applies to scientific enquiry (the research). The evidence is the results of experiments designed to measure or support – or call into question – a scientific hypothesis, or theory. The evidence must be laid out in line with normal scientific standards applicable to the field of study. It may also encompass numerical analysis of results by statistical tests used to support the theory. All these elements will be taught to you as part of your undergraduate research course and will help you understand how to use published evidence.

How do I look for evidence?

The evidence may come from a variety of sources (see Useful resources). Some may come from the personal experience of qualified chiropractors (case studies), some from the opinions of acknowledged experts in the field (anecdotal evidence or personal communication) and other evidence may come from specific studies or projects designed to answer a clinical question, such as cohort studies and randomised controlled clinical trials (RCTs).

Evidence from small studies can be of limited value, but this value can be increased significantly if all the small studies are collated together and analysed to give a 'consensus answer'. This is the basis of systematic review and 'meta-analysis', which is a form of collective analysis. Each of these evidence sources has a value in its own right, but some types have a larger impact and carry a greater weight of opinion than others. This gives rise to the so-called 'hierarchy of evidence' (See Figure 16.1). The hierarchy is a classification that shows the relative strength of types of evidence: systematic reviews, for example, are at the top of the 'pile' while personal communication (perhaps a chat over a cup of tea) is at the bottom. This is useful when evaluating the evidence for a particular problem or question.

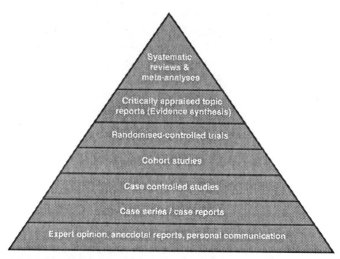

Figure 16.1. The hierarchy of evidence

What is evidence-based practice?

Evidence-based practice (EBP) is probably one of the most frequently used terms you will hear during your undergraduate career and throughout your postgraduate practice. The term was first coined for the medical profession and has now grown to encompass many of the clinical disciplines.

Definition

Evidence-based practice has been defined as '*the explicit use of the best clinically relevant evidence in making decisions about the care of individual patients*' (Sackett, 1997).

'I find that evidence-based practice, basically, is all about "joining up the dots" between research and clinical practice, including the patients' expectations. I try to reinforce this with my chiropractic students at an early stage of study.

Many students are surprised that 'what the patient wants' forms part of good evidence-based practice, but patient expectation is crucial to the process. Regardless of what you, as a qualified practitioner, might regard as the best treatment approach, the patient has the final say in accepting, modifying or rejecting your plan. Patients' expectations hinge on their values (philosophical or religious beliefs), their concerns (clinical and non-clinical, such as finance and time) and their expectations (time taken to 'cure'). Expectations have a major impact on results and the published literature is full of patient attitude surveys to support this.

Good chiropractors use their clinical expertise to plan patient treatments, but they also use current research evidence, as they are not mutually exclusive. The evidence used is not restricted to systematic reviews or RCTs, but also includes relevant case studies to illustrate important clinical points. Since the application of scientific evidence plays such a critical role in the clinical decision-making process, students in any healthcare discipline should learn and use evidence-based skills during their study. The development of these skills includes research theory, evidence gathering coupled with fundamental literature searching and critical appraisal skills (see Chapters 10 and 11). As a student, you should subsequently be able to integrate and apply these skills to clinical decision-making.

The evidence base and chiropractic

Your perception of EBP will translate to 'evidence-based chiropractic', or EBC, as you move through your career. EBC is simply a specific variant of evidence-based medicine (EBM). It has the same steps and principles, but is modelled around questions specific to chiropractic as a treatment. Just as EBM has been accepted into the medical profession and EBP has been adopted by many of the healthcare professions, EBC has been embraced by the vast majority of the chiropractic profession. The basic tenants of EBC are taught at all colleges offering chiropractic training.

This is important for the profession to advance alongside other mainstream healthcare professions. EBC should be a preferred choice in practice as it offers the best *opportunities* to deliver high-quality results in patient care. This is achieved, simply, by using those practices that have been shown to benefit patients, according to the research evidence, while avoiding those which have not. EBC must be used judiciously, however, in conjunction with your clinical experience and judgement, the clinical circumstances of the presenting patient and the personal preferences of the patient.

Benefits to the profession

EBC provides many benefits for the chiropractic profession, for example, it can help you gain a much better relationship with the medical profession as a whole. Chiropractic has made huge inroads into public acceptance over the last 20 years or so. Due to its holistic approach to treating neuro-musculoskeletal conditions, it is highly regarded by the public and enjoys one of the highest levels of patient satisfaction with positive outcomes.

The current healthcare system in the UK dictates that the General Practitioner (GP) remains the gateway to many referrals (both NHS and private). Changing the way GPs think about chiropractic is key to increasing the referral of patients for treatment. Doctors already have a good professional relationship with other healthcare professions based upon effective communication and this is where chiropractors can alter perceptions (see Chapter 2).

Top tip

Many GPs express a keen wish to understand more about the chiropractic profession, and that is where you, as part of new generation of chiropractors, can change the patterns of GP referral by communicating with the medical profession on its own terms.

There have been several research studies which show that good levels of communication between healthcare professions have a beneficial effect on patient care but, paradoxically, the levels of communication between GPs and chiropractors has been quite poor. Past surveys of GPs have found that chiropractors who do communicate with GPs tend to be dogmatic in their approach and sometimes fail to provide sufficient evidence for treatment. With the current planned changes in the healthcare system in the UK, especially around provision of musculoskeletal services, there has never been a better time for chiropractors to become key players in primary healthcare in this country. How can this be achieved? By contributing to, and improving on, the evidence base for chiropractic treatment and by forging credible and professional alliances with the medical profession.

Case study: Barriers between GPs and chiropractors

This is an example from one of a number of student studies into the referral patterns of GPs and how the chiropractic profession could increase the rate of onward referral from them. The GP is the gateway to onward referral in the NHS and consequently their opinion can influence that of the general public. Although awareness of chiropractic among GPs may be high, only 33% preferred chiropractic referral for manipulative therapy. The use of complementary and alternative medicine (CAM), including chiropractic, is rising and so integrating CAM and mainstream medicine into a framework could prove to be an important factor in public health in the future. By investigating the barriers to GPs referral to chiropractors, an understanding of the attitudes of GPs, assessment of their knowledge of the chiropractic profession and their likelihood to refer in the future could be identified and help provide a solution where both sectors of healthcare can work symbiotically.

Why is there not more evidence-based chiropractic research?

There are two main reasons why EBC remains distinct when compared with other evidence-based research models, and you should bear these in mind when considering or discussing the volume of EBC in the field:

1. Chiropractic interventions do not always lend themselves easily to investigation by the standard medical research design methods created to test new drugs or surgical techniques, for example. Also, chiropractors often employ a number of different techniques in the treatment of a single patient and this can provide a dilemma in the analysis of results.

2. Chiropractic is fairly low in the pecking order for significant levels of research funding, and limited funding hampers the conduct of major pieces of work. Research is expensive and pharmaceutical companies, for example, have huge financial resources in contrast. As the evidence base for chiropractic increases, however, it will be easier to construct cases to apply for major UK grants for more research.

The current key evidence

Chiropractic has been shown to be a very safe form of treatment with good outcomes and, in spite of these constraints, the evidence base in chiropractic has grown significantly over the last 15 to 20 years. A number of recent systematic reviews and clinical trial reports show that chiropractic provides good value, both clinically and in terms of cost-effectiveness, as an intervention for many conditions. Both the Cochrane Collaboration and the National Institute for Clinical Excellence (NICE) have issued reports and guidelines (see Chapter 2) showing that chiropractic is effective for many musculoskeletal conditions. The available evidence base for chiropractic shows it to be of value in managing a variety of conditions such as types of:

- Low back pain
- Radiating pain
- Whiplash injuries
- Neck pain
- Headaches

Programme modules and the dissertation

You are introduced to the process of research in a systematic way during your degree and *dissertation* is not as scary as it sounds! A systematic approach to your research and the completion of a good dissertation involves:

1. **Identification of a research problem:** providing a general statement of the problem or reasons for engaging in the research.

2. **Literature review:** investigating what is already known about the subject area and what light this throws on your reasons for researching the area.

3. **Specific research issue:** this is your hypothesis – what you want to prove.

4. **Data collection:** this is collecting the evidence to answer your problem. The modes of data collection vary depending on the type of research undertaken and the types of method design employed.

5. **Analysing and interpreting the data:** this is what most students fear – the statistics. What does your data actually tell you about your project?

6. **Reporting and evaluating research:** writing up your findings and telling everyone what you have discovered. This can be a very rewarding part of the process and you may have your work accepted at a national or international conference.

You should regard this as an evolving and fluid process rather than being completely fixed. For most current chiropractic programmes, the whole of your 'research journey' will take place over a four-year period and involve three exercises: the research proposal, the research protocol and the research dissertation.

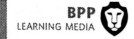

Undertaking research year-by-year

Chiropractic programmes are all different in the way they approach research in the curriculum, but there are some basic elements that are common throughout. Here is an example of a standard approach to reassure you that you will be shown how to build gradually to the final product.

Initially, you will be taught the theoretical and background aspects of research, providing you with some basic knowledge to underpin future years. It will most likely be lecture-based covering topics such as the place of research in clinical practice, research paradigms (the philosophies behind research), basic method design and how to search for, read and evaluate scientific literature.

Next, you will build on this knowledge, and be introduced to what data is and how to analyse it. You also start to learn how to critically appraise the scientific literature you read, which is essential for the proper practice of EBC. More importantly, however, you start to formulate your future research project in the form of a research proposal document. This is, essentially, a statement of your research question that you would like to answer, followed by an outline plan of how you think you can achieve this (your method and analysis) and how feasible your study is.

Research questions can be encouraged in brainstorming sessions with lecturers and fellow students. Previous dissertations may leave unanswered questions that beg a follow-on study or they might prompt a slightly different line of enquiry. The research question you pose at this point might not be the final version for your dissertation – it can undergo many iterations and modifications as you pass through the various elements of the research course.

Proposal and protocol stages

You will then write a proposal document which will need to be reviewed and approved. As part of the process, you can expect to justify what the value your research will be; for example, how might it improve patient care or advance the chiropractic profession. There are two clear threads of chiropractic research that define the routes of study: the first is quality from both the patient and research perspective and the second is outcome measures (or how you will measure the effectiveness of your research).

Following approval of the proposal, you will gain more experience of critical appraisal, statistical analysis and literature searching. It also is the time you complete your research protocol. The protocol is a formal document that represents a planning guide, or 'instruction book', that starts the process of your research and data collection. In most cases it is a natural progression from the proposal document produced in the second year. It is a detailed document stating your research question, providing a detailed background literature review, a methodology (including how you plan to analyse the collected data) and some assessment of the possible outcomes. Preparing the protocol can be a bit exasperating to a novice researcher but the document does need to be detailed. It is the assessment document for ethical review and must confirm that your project will meet all the tenets of common decency and political correctness! Once you have passed this hurdle, the next part is relatively straightforward.

Final dissertation

Then you move on to actually collecting data for your final dissertation. This is the exciting time. The dissertation tells the story of your research: from setting the scene (the introduction); through showing the extent of current knowledge (the literature review); explaining how you undertook the study and who you used as participants (the methods) and then showing what your study found (the results). Finally, you explain how your study links with the current knowledge (the discussion), before providing a clear statement that places your work in the context of current theory and how it applies to practice (the conclusions).

You may also be asked to give a presentation of your findings to your peer group and other students. This can be invaluable for a number of reasons. First, it can help you crystallise your thoughts before you write up your study and, second, it allows you to rehearse arguments and theories and test them with colleagues in an informal environment. Third, this process gives you valuable experience in presentation skills. These may be vital for you in the future, especially if your work is successful in submissions to conferences and you find yourself presenting to an international audience!

If this all sounds a bit daunting, do not be put off – the research and teaching staff are there to help you at each stage. Although the research project must be your own work, you are assigned a supervisor to advise and guide you (usually at the protocol stage after submission of the proposal). You need to have a good relationship with your supervisor and communicate with them regularly. This person will be your mentor: helping you to develop ideas; advising you if you are straying from your question; guiding you out of trouble (academically speaking!) and helping you write up by proof-reading your work. Beware, however, the supervisor is there as a critical friend and not someone to do the work for you.

Chapter summary

Completing a research project gives you a much deeper understanding of what you are studying. The experience will help you develop and hone many skills necessary in your new field of work, including the skills of lifelong learning which is essential if you are to improve your practice for the benefit of patients. It will also show others that you can complete a major piece of academic work (and you will have the evidence to prove it!).

For the chiropractic profession to continue to grow from strength to strength, evidence-based research in this field must be enhanced and extended. Undertaking and implementing the types of research that are needed will require a great commitment (from students and clinicians alike) to the basic science, clinical expertise and critical thinking that underpins the profession – more so than ever before. This is how the profession will move on and why research is now such a key area of study in all chiropractic programmes.

Key points

- Research is the systematic seeking of evidence to answer a particular question. This may involve literature reviews and / or experimentation.

- Chiropractic research modules provide you with the necessary skills to think and appraise evidence in a critical manner – both while studying and as a practitioner.

- Evidence is the data used to support or reject a theory.

- The evidence base is the research available to help you make clinical decisions for the benefit of patients.

- Improving the chiropractic evidence base and also communications between healthcare professionals is an obligation for all qualified practitioners.

Useful resources

Anglo-European College of Chiropractic – research at the AECC:
www.aecc.ac.uk/research

ChiroACCESS clinical review pages: www.chiroaccess.com

Chiro Org – Chiropractic Research: www.chiro.org/research

Dynamic Chiropractic research review pages:
www.chiropracticresearch.org

McTimoney College of Chiropractic – research pages:
www.mctimoney-college.ac.uk/about/research

University of Glamorgan chiropractic research:
http://chiropractic.research.glam.ac.uk

References

Sackett, DL. Evidence-based medicine. *Semin Perinatol* 1997 Feb;
21(1): 3–5.

Index

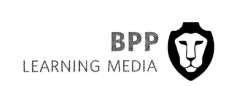